New Developments in Medical Research

nova
Medicine & Health
New York

New Developments in Medical Research

Botulinum Toxin: Therapeutic Uses, Procedures and Efficacy
James C. Lark (Editor)
2022. ISBN: 978-1-68507-817-1 (Hardcover)
2022. ISBN: 978-1-68507-826-3 (eBook)

Evidence-Based Medicine: From the Clinician and Educator Perspective
Sowdhamini Wallace, DO, MS (Editor)
Ganga Gokulakrishnan, MD, MS (Editor)
2022. ISBN: 978-1-68507-546-0 (Hardcover)
2022. ISBN: 978-1-68507-700-6 (eBook)

COVID-19 by Cases: A Pandemic Review
Sujanthy S. Rajaram, MD, MPH, FACP, FAASM, FCCM (Editor)
Anthony Longo, MD (Editor)
Nicole Burak, MD (Editor)
2021. ISBN: 978-1-68507-099-1 (Hardcover)
2021. ISBN: 978-1-68507-262-9 (eBook)

Respiratory Care in Non Invasive Mechanical Ventilatory Support: Principles and Practice
Antonio M. Esquinas, M.D, PhD (Editor)
Mohammed Alahmari, PhD (Editor)
2021. ISBN: 978-1-53619-702-0 (Hardcover)
2021. ISBN: 978-1-53619-902-4 (eBook)

Platelet-Rich Plasma: Myths vs. Reality, Health Effects, and Risks
Pietro Gentile, MD, PhD (Author)
2021. ISBN: 978-1-53619-722-8 (eBook)

More information about this series can be found at
https://novapublishers.com/product-category/series/new-developments-in-medical-research/

Mila Maidarti, Hariyono Winarto,
Chyntia Olivia Maurine Jasirwan,
Eka Dian Safitri and
Virna Dwi Oktariana
Editors

The 6th Annual International Conference and Exhibition on Indonesian Medical Education and Research Institute (6th ICE on IMERI) 2021

nova
Medicine & Health
New York

https://doi.org/10.52305/RLQB3573

Library of Congress Cataloging-in-Publication Data

ISBN: 978-1-68507-925-3

Published by Nova Science Publishers, Inc. † New York

Contents

Preface

The 6th Annual International Conference and Exhibition on IMERI 2021 (ICE on IMERI 2021) is the annual international medical conference held by The Indonesian Medical Education and Research Institute. The 6th ICE on IMERI 2021 addresses the theme "Biomedical Research and Primary Care Transformation: The Potential Issue in the Post Pandemic Era." This conference was held on November 6-7 & 13-14, 2021, virtually.

This conference brings together a multi-disciplinary group of all professions involved in the field, including academicians to policymakers, researchers, clinicians, technocrats, and other related disciplines, to present and exchange ideas relating to medical science and presenting some outstanding speakers coming from Indonesia, Japan, Australia, The United Kingdom, Thailand, Italy, USA, and Singapore.

The 6th ICE on IMERI 2021 provides some programs consisting of a main symposium and workshops. The main symposium consists of 9 keynote lectures and 22 concurrent sessions delivered by experts experienced in healthcare, professionals, and researchers around the world. There are 12 workshops held by IMERI research clusters comprising Center of e-Learning, Drug Development (DDRC), Center for Sports and Exercise Studies, Medical Technology, Center for Sports and Exercise Studies: Human Cancer (HCRC), Bioinformatics, Human Nutrition (HNRC), Human Genetic (HGRC), Metabolic Disorder, Cardiovascular and Aging (MVA), Writing Center, and Center for Sports and Exercise Studies.

We would like to thank the organizing committee, editorial boards, editorial assistants, and reviewers. They have given immense contribution in evaluating articles and providing essential suggestions for authors to enhance the quality of their articles.

Mila Maidarti
General Chair

Acknowledgements

Foremost, we would like to express our gratitude to the publication committee of the 6th ICE on IMERI 2021, who had supported the Proceeding Publication in Nova Science Publishers, Inc.

We thank all Editorial Boards, Dr. dr. Hariyono Winarto, Sp.OG(K); dr. Chyntia Olivia Maurine Jasirwan; Sp.PD, Ph.D., dr. Eka Dian Safitri, Sp.THT-KL; and Dr. dr. Virna Dwi Oktariana, SpM(K), reviewed and evaluated each research article and all Editorial Assistants, dr. Fiona Esmeralda., MM; dr. Nur Eulis Pujiastuti Nahdiyat, M.Res; dr. Aly Lamuri, MSc; dr. Daniel Martin Simadibrata, M. Res; and dr. Naivedh Bhat, BmedSci for comments that greatly improved the articles.

We would like to show our gratitude to Karomah Widianingsih, S.Hum, and Indiana Tarziah, S.E, who had provided significant contributions in managing all research articles. We would like also thank Nova Science Publishers, Inc. for publishing our conference articles.

Chapter 1

The Impact of Sociodemographic Factors on Knowledge, Attitude, and Behaviour of Health and Non-Health Science Students for COVID-19 Prevention in Indonesia

Monika Herliana[1], Lubna Djafar[1], Bagas Ariffandi[1], Eric Ferdinand[1], Shakila Zuleika Putri[2], Muhammad Fakhri Prayitno[1], Bagus Amartya Yudhananto[3], Kamila Nurul Najmi[4] and Retno Asti Werdhani[1,*]

[1]Faculty of Medicine, Universitas Indonesia, Jakarta, Indonesia
[2]Faculty of Medicine Universitas Airlangga, Surabaya, Indonesia
[3]Faculty of Medicine Universitas Gadjah Mada, Daerah Istimewa Yogyakarta, Indonesia
[4]Faculty of Medicine Universitas Sebelas Maret, Surakarta, Indonesia

Abstract

Background: Sufficient knowledge, a good attitude and good behaviour are essential to overcome the COVID-19 pandemic. This chapter identifies the different levels of knowledge, attitudes and behaviours of COVID-19 prevention between health and non-health science students with different socio-demographic and socioeconomic factors. *Methods:* A cross-sectional study was conducted at 14 universities in major cities of Indonesia. The 793 samples were obtained through a convenience sampling technique using an adapted online questionnaire. A descriptive and bivariate analysis was performed using the Statistical Package for the

* Corresponding Author's Email: retno.asti@ui.ac.id.

In: The 6th Annual International Conference …
Editors: M. Maidarti, H. Winarto, C. O. M. Jasirwan et al.
ISBN: 978-1-68507-925-3

Social Sciences (SPSS) programme version 20. *Results:* The majority of the respondents were female health science students aged < 20 years, who were residents of Java and had a household income ≥IDR 3,500,000. Of the respondents, 54.7% had sufficient knowledge of COVID-19, 73.9% had a good attitude, and 74.1% showed good behaviour. Health science students had higher knowledge scores ($p < .001$) and better behaviour ($p = .012$). Female students and those with a household income ≥IDR 3,500,000 had significantly better attitudes and behaviours ($p = .011$ and $p < .001$). A significant relationship exists between both knowledge and behaviour ($p = .047$) and between attitude and behaviour ($p < .001$), while knowledge and attitude have no significant relationship ($p = .178$). *Conclusion:* There are different levels of knowledge, attitude and behaviour regarding COVID-19 prevention among health and non-health science students, genders and people with different household incomes. Knowledge and attitude levels are related to COVID-19 prevention behaviour, while knowledge and attitude level are unrelated.

Keywords: knowledge, attitude, behaviour, COVID-19, students

Introduction

Coronavirus, commonly known as COVID-19, is a disease caused by severe acute respiratory syndrome coronavirus 2 (SARS-CoV 2) and is estimated to have first appeared in March 2019 in China as a new coronavirus disease, which now has a major impact on all sectors of life globally [1]. A World Health Organization (WHO) report released on April 4, 2021 claimed there were 130,459,184 cases and 2,842,325 deaths due to COVID-19 worldwide [2]. The data also show that the number of positive cases of COVID-19 in Indonesia has reached 1,527,524, with the number of new death cases and cumulative deaths being 878 and 41,242, respectively. Indonesia is one of the countries in Southeast Asia that still reported a high number of new cases until the end of the second week of September 2020 [2]. Some of the effects of this pandemic in the short term are the high rate of layoffs, which led to increased unemployment and decreased productivity, industry losses, and hotel and tourism business restrictions [3].

One strategy for dealing with a pandemic is to implement a protocol that prevents the spread of COVID-19 related to setting standards for the use of personal protective equipment, implementing large-scale social restrictions (PSBB) and adapting to new life habits [3]. Even though the Indonesian government has established this policy, many people have continued to disobey the regulations, carried out many activities outside the home, taken trips to various places, and returned to their hometowns without proper protection [4]. Although recently the COVID-19 vaccine has been developed and used in the community, not all groups of people have received the vaccine, and further research on immunological and safety aspects is still needed [5, 6]. Before we can eradicate COVID-19 with vaccines, other preventive measures are still needed to inhibit the rate of increase in COVID-19 cases. Health knowledge, attitude and behaviour are among the important factors related to disease prevention. Therefore, people's knowledge, attitudes and behaviour are vital in determining the success of government policies to tackle the COVID-19 pandemic [4].

As an educated community group, students can become role models for the community in carrying out the regulations set by the government [7]. Ideally, health science students should have a better level of knowledge than most others about how to prevent and control COVID-19 due to their exposure to information about health in daily life, so they tend to have a good attitude [8]. According to a systematic review by Ernawati et al., (2021), preventive behaviour against COVID-19 is positively correlated with the knowledge and attitudes of each community [9]. However, knowledge cannot always determine a person's behaviour. According to the theory of the health belief model, conditions under serious threat, vulnerability and the benefits of an action determine whether a person is like to take preventive action [10]. Also, as conflicts remain between the results of several studies examining the relationships between knowledge, attitudes and behaviour against COVID-19, which have been carried out in several places in Indonesia, further research is needed to confirm the results of previous research [8, 11-13].

Therefore, this chapter determines the distribution of knowledge levels with students' attitudes and behaviours and compares the levels of knowledge, attitude and behaviour between groups of people with different socio-demographic and socioeconomic backgrounds. This research also compares behaviours of health and non-health science students in carrying out the protocol that has been established by the Indonesian government to prevent the transmission of COVID-19.

Materials and Methods

The study was conducted from January to April 2021 as cross-sectional research. Primary data were obtained through a Google Forms questionnaire, which was distributed through social media platforms by Center for Indonesian Medical Students' Activities (CIMSA) representatives. The target population of this chapter was active health science and non-health science students from 14 universities in major cities of Indonesia that have an established Standing Committee on Research Exchange (SCORE) CIMSA local structure. Students were recruited specifically from Java and Sumatra, which are the most populated islands in Indonesia and have had the highest numbers of COVID-19 cases in Indonesia. Samples were obtained using the convenience sampling method. The number of samples was calculated using analytical cross-sectional sample formulas with a 95% confidence interval and 80% power research. The inclusion criteria were students aged 18-25 years who had agreed to fill out the Google Forms questionnaire voluntarily, while the exclusion criteria were students who could not access our questionnaire.

The knowledge section of the questionnaire used in this chapter was adapted from studies by Zhong et al. and Olum et al., while the attitude and behaviour section was derived from a public survey in the COVID-19 pandemic by the National Central Bureau of Statistics [14-16]. Collected variables included gender, age, domain/area/residency, household income, and knowledge, attitude and behaviour scores for COVID-19 preventions. Knowledge scores were measured through nine true/false questions while both attitude and behaviour scores were determined as an average of six Likert scale items, ranging from 1 (never) to 10 (always). The total internal consistency (Cronbach's alpha) of the questionnaire was 0.94. Data were analysed descriptively and analytically using the Statistical Package for Social Sciences (SPSS) programme for Windows version 20 and presented as frequency distribution with percentages for categorical variables and median and range values for numerical variables. Knowledge, attitude and behaviour scores were classified into two groups, which were scores with values less than 8 and scores with values 8 and above. The bivariate analysis for proportional differences among groups was done using the chi-square test. This study obtained ethical approval from the Health Research Ethics Committee of Faculty of Medicine Universitas Sebelas Maret with ethical clearance number 03/UN27.06.6.1/KEPK/EC.2021. All data presented in this chapter were obtained with the consent of the respondents.

Results

Characteristics of Respondents Based on Socio-Demographic Factors

Of 802 respondents, 9 were excluded due to incomplete or missing data, giving a final total of 793 students. This number met the minimum sample size requirement with more than 80% research power. The majority of respondents were aged below 20 years (50.4%), with ages ranging from 18 to 24 years old and a median age of 19 years old. More respondents were female (76%) and were health science students (54.4%). Most of the respondents originated from Java Island (85%) and had a household income above Rp 3,500,000 (69.2%) (Table 1).

Table 1. Respondents based on socio-demographic factors (n = 793)

Variables	**n (%)**	**Median (Min-Max)**
Age (years old)		19 (18-24)
<20 years old	400 (50.4)	
≥20 years old	393 (49.6)	
Gender		
Male	190 (24)	
Female	603 (76)	
Domain/Area/Residency		
Java	674 (85)	
Outside of Java	119 (15)	
Household income		
Below Rp 3,500,000	244 (30.8)	
Rp 3,500,000 and above	549 (69.2)	
Study field		
Health sciences	431 (54.4)	
Non-health sciences	362 (45.6)	

Characteristics of Respondents Based on their Knowledge, Attitude and Behaviour towards COVID-19

None of the scores for knowledge, attitude or behaviour showed a normal data distribution. Thus, results are presented in the form of median and ranges. The respondents' knowledge of COVID-19 was found to be generally sufficient, with the majority scoring 8 or above (54.7%). Accordingly, most respondents showed a good attitude towards COVID-19 prevention and frequently practiced measures (73.9% and 74.1%, respectively), as represented by an average score of 8 or above (Table 2).

Table 2. Respondents' knowledge, attitude and behaviour towards COVID-19 (n =793)

Variables	n (%)	Median (Min-Max)
Knowledge (max score 10)		8.88 (2.22–10)
Score below 8	359 (45.3)	
Score 8 and above	434 (54.7)	
Attitude (max score 10)		9 (1–10)
Poor	207 (26.1)	
Good	586 (73.9)	
Behaviour (max score 10)		9 (1–10)
Never/seldom	205 (25.9)	
Frequent	588 (74.1)	

Relationship between Knowledge and Health and Non-Health Sciences Students

Health sciences students had a significantly higher number of good knowledge scores for COVID-19 prevention measures than non-health sciences students (p = <.001). However, no significant difference was found in knowledge scores between age group, gender, residency and household income (Table 3).

Table 3. Relationship between knowledge and socio-demographic and socio-economic factors (n = 793)

Variables	Knowledge Score		*P*-value
	Below 8 N (%)	8 and above N (%)	
Age			
<20 years old	171 (42.8)	229 (57.3)	
>20 years old	188 (47.8)	205 (52.2)	.150
Gender			
Male	85 (44.7)	105 (55.3)	
Female	274 (45.4)	329 (54.6)	.865
Domain/Area/Residency			
Java	300 (44.5)	374 (55.5)	
Outside of Java	59 (49.6)	60 (50.4)	.306
Household income			
Below Rp 3,500,000	119 (48.8)	125 (51.2)	
Rp 3,500,000 and above	240 (47.3)	309 (56.3)	.187
Study field			
Health sciences	148 (34.3)	283 (65.7)	
Non-health sciences	211 (58.3)	151 (41.7)	<.001

Relationship between Attitude and Socio-Demographic and Socio-Economic Factors

Female respondents had a significantly higher number of good attitude scores towards COVID-19 prevention than males (*p* = .011). A significantly better attitude score could also be observed in respondents with a monthly household income of Rp 3,500,000 and above (*p* <.001) (Table 4).

Table 4. Relationship between Attitude and Socio-Demographic and Socio-Economic Factors (n = 793)

Variables	**Attitude Score**		***P*-value**
	Poor N (%)	**Good N (%)**	
Age			
<20 years old	96 (24)	304 (76)	
>20 years old	111 (28.2)	282 (71.8)	.174
Gender			
Male	63 (33.2)	127 (66.8)	
Female	144 (23.9)	459 (76.1)	.011
Domain/Area/Residency			
Java	175 (26)	499 (74)	
Outside of Java	32 (26,9)	87 (73,1)	.832
Household income			
Below Rp 3,500,000	86 (35.2)	158 (64.8)	
Rp 3,500,000 and above	121 (22)	428 (78)	<.001
Study field			
Health sciences	101 (23.4)	330 (76.6)	
Non-health sciences	106 (29.3)	256 (70.7)	.062

Relationship between Behaviour and Socio-Demographic and Socio-Economic Factors

In line with our findings for attitude, female respondents and those with higher household incomes were also more likely to achieve good or 'frequent' behaviour scores (*p* < .001) for practicing COVID-19 prevention measures. Health sciences students were also more likely to have good behaviour than students from non-health sciences fields (*p* = .012) (Table 5).

Table 5. Relationship between behaviour and socio-demographic and socio-economic factors (n = 793)

Variables	Behaviour Score		*P*-value
	Never/seldom N (%)	**Frequent N (%)**	
Age			
<20 years old	97 (24.3)	303 (75.8)	
>20 years old	108 (27.5)	285 (72.5)	.299
Gender			
Male	71 (37.4)	119 (62.6)	
Female	134 (22.2)	469 (77.8)	<.001
Domain/Area/Residency			
Java	166 (24.6)	508 (75.4)	
Outside of Java	39 (32.8)	80 (67.2)	.061
Household income			
Below Rp 3,500,000	84 (34.4)	160 (65.6)	
Rp 3,500,000 and above	121 (22)	428 (78)	<.001
Study field			
Health sciences	96 (22.3)	335 (77.7)	
Non-health sciences	109 (25.9)	253 (69.9)	.012

Distribution of Respondents' Responses on Knowledge, Attitude and Behaviour

The highest number of incorrect answers were found on question number 2 about the common symptoms of COVID-19 and question number 5 about modes of viral transmission (Table 6).

Generally, the majority of respondents achieved good attitude and behaviour scores (Tables 7 and 8). The least practiced preventive measure is minimal 1-metre physical distancing, as seen in Table 8.

From Table 9, it can be interpreted that students with frequent COVID-19 prevention behaviour were more likely to have a sufficient level of knowledge (56.8%) compared to students who never or seldom performed behaviours to prevent COVID-19 (48.8%). The proportion difference was statistically significant ($p = .047$).

In line with our findings regarding knowledge and behaviour relationships, students who frequently practiced COVID-19 prevention behaviours were also more likely to have a good attitude (87.9%) compared to students who never or seldom engaged in COVID-19 prevention (33.7.8%). The difference in proportion was statistically significant ($p < .001$). However, no significant relationship was found between knowledge and attitude scores ($p = .914$) (Table 10).

Table 6. Distribution of respondents' responses on knowledge (n = 793)

Questions	Correct Answer	Incorrect Answer
The main symptoms of COVID-19 include fever, fatigue, dry cough and myalgia. (TRUE)	707 (89.2%)	86 (10.8%)
Symptoms of nasal congestion, runny nose and sneezing are less common in COVID-19 than with the common cold. (TRUE)	439 (54.5%)	361 (45.5%)
There is currently no effective treatment for COVID-19. However, early symptom management and supportive therapy can improve patients' recovery. (TRUE)	719 (90.7%)	74 (9.3%)
Not all patients with COVID-19 develop severe symptoms. Only the elderly, people with chronic illnesses and people with obesity are more likely to have a severe illness. (TRUE)	643 (81.1%)	150 (18.9%)
Consumption of and direct contact with wild animals can cause COVID-19 infection. (FALSE)	452 (57.0%)	343 (43.0%)
People with COVID-19 cannot transmit the virus to other people if they do not have fever symptoms. (FALSE)	699 (88.1%)	94 (11.9%)
The COVID-19 virus spreads through respiratory droplets. (TRUE)	724 (91.3%)	69 (8.7%)
Isolation and management of infected patients are effective ways to reduce viral transmissions. (TRUE)	772 (97.4%)	21 (2.6%)
People who have a history of contact with COVID-19 patients are required to immediately self-isolate. The general observation time is 14 days. (TRUE)	772 (97.4%)	21 (2.6%)

Table 7. Distribution of respondents' responses on attitude (n = 793)

Questions	Score 8 and Above	Score Below 8
How effectively does wearing masks prevent the COVID-19 infection?	618 (77.9%)	175 (22.1%)
How effectively does washing your hands with soap for at least 20 seconds prevent COVID-19 infection?	610 (76.9%)	183 (23.1%)
How effectively does using hand sanitiser prevent COVID-19 infection?	581 (73.3%)	212 (26.7%)
How effectively does avoiding handshakes and other physical contact prevent COVID-19 infection?	633 (79.8%)	160 (20.2%)
How effectively does avoiding crowds prevent COVID-19 infection?	655 (82.6%)	138 (17.4%)
How effectively does 1-metre physical distancing prevent COVID-19 infection?	600 (75.7%)	193 (24.3%)

Table 8. Distribution of respondents' response on behaviour (n = 793)

Questions	Frequent	Never/Seldom
In the last seven days, how often have you worn a mask when you are out?	684 (86.3%)	109 (13.7%)
In the last seven days, how often have you washed your hands with soap for at least 20 seconds when you are out?	575 (72.5%)	218 (27.5%)
In the last seven days, how often have you used hand sanitiser when you are out?	614 (77.4%)	179 (22.6%)
In the last seven days, how often have you avoided handshakes or another physical contact when you are out?	600 (75.7%)	193 (24.3%)
In the last seven days, how often have you avoided a crowded place when you are out?	575 (72.5%)	218 (27.5%)
In the last seven days, how often have you kept a 1-metre physical distance when you are out?	537 (67.7%)	256 (32.3%)

Table 9. Relationship attitude and behaviour towards knowledge

	Knowledge Score		
	Below 8	**8 and above**	***P*-value**
Attitude			
Poor	102 (49.3)	105 (50.7)	
Good	257 (43.9)	329 (56.1)	.178
Behaviour			
Never/seldom	105 (51.2)	100 (48.8)	
Frequent	254 (43.2)	334 (56.8)	.047

Table 10. Relationship knowledge and behaviour towards attitude

	Attitude Scale		
	Poor N (%)	**Good N (%)**	**P-value**
Knowledge			
Score <8	102 (28.4)	257 (71.6)	.194
Score ≥8	105 (24.2)	329 (75.8)	
Behaviour			
Never/seldom	136 (66.3)	69 (33.7)	<.001
Frequent	71 (12.1)	517 (87.9)	

Discussion

Our results show that most students have adequate knowledge of COVID-19 prevention. This result aligns with similar studies conducted with students in India, Jordan and China, which showed that more than 80% of undergraduate students were aware of the main symptoms of COVID-19 and that, at the time of this research, there was no clinically effective treatment for COVID-19 [17-19]. In particular, Maheshwari et al., (2020) used a very similar set of questions to test for knowledge, with similar results to ours [17].

Regarding attitude, our study shows that most students have appropriate attitudes regarding COVID-19 health protocol, with more than 75% of respondents agreeing with common health protocol acts, such as wearing a mask, washing their hands, and avoiding physical contact and proximities. This finding agrees with the results from a similar study in Jordan, although notably, their result suggests a smaller percentage of students agreed that wearing a mask helped contain the pandemic when compared to our data [18]. This difference might be due to differences in culture and information between Indonesia and Jordan.

Notably, our study indicates that age is not correlated with knowledge, attitude or behaviour towards COVID-19. This result contrasts with several previous studies in Indonesia, which reported that older age is associated with better knowledge, probably due to more knowledge gained in the past and an increased ability to apprehend the information [4, 12, 20-21]. Nonetheless, our study corresponds with a study by Prihati et al., (2020), which showed that no correlation existed between age and COVID-19 preventive behavior [22]. From these comparisons, we consider that the narrow age range in our study likely affected our result.

Gender difference was found to correlate with attitude and behaviour. In our study, female students had significantly better attitudes and behaviour compared to male students. This result supports the findings of several previous studies [21, 23-24]. Females are known to be concerned more about health issues in general. Therefore, women considered COVID-19 to be a serious health problem and are associated with lower COVID-19 mortality compared to males because of better compliance with public health rules [21, 23-25]. Furthermore, in contrast to millennial males who use the internet to obtain information about sports and weather, females tend to use the internet to obtain health information. As this research topic is more interesting for females, it also explains the reason for a larger number of female respondents in our study [26]. However, our study contradicted the findings of Prihati et al., (2020), who reported no correlation between gender and behaviour towards COVID-19 [22].

Based on our study, although it is not significantly associated with a better attitude, health science students are associated with better knowledge and behaviour. This finding is supported by Usman et al., (2020), who showed that

Indonesian health science students have good knowledge in preventing COVID-19 transmission in Indonesia. At the same time, our study contradicts Usman et al., (2020) in terms of attitude [8]. To our knowledge, research and literature that compared health science students' and non-health science students' knowledge, attitude and behaviour towards COVID-19 prevention are rarely available. We suggest that easier access and more exposure to health information, especially about COVID-19 prevention, may improve the knowledge of the health science students as well as non-health science students towards COVID-19.

Our results reveal that no significant difference existed between students' knowledge, attitude and behaviour towards COVID-19 health protocol within and outside Java. Although this result differed from the monitoring survey published by the Indonesian COVID-19 Task Force in March 2021, which showed better protocol compliance in Java compared to Sumatra, the survey did not compare the results using analytical statistics [27]. To our knowledge, this chapter is the first to compare the knowledge, attitude and behaviour within and outside Java. From this result, we inferred that there is no difference in the information and education received inside Java and outside Java. Nonetheless, further research is needed to confirm these results.

Income is an important factor that influences attitude and behaviour. According to our study, a higher income correlates with better attitude and behaviour. A similar result was found by Wonok et al., (2020), who also suggested that income influences the capability of people to access more information and facilities [20]. Mujani et al., (2020) showed similar results, suggesting a higher income was associated with higher education and thus had better financial durability to temporarily stop doing the activity or working outdoors for a while [24].

We also found a significant difference between knowledge and behaviour. Students with good knowledge were related to having frequent behaviour for COVID-19 prevention. As expected from the health belief model, perceived knowledge of the COVID-19 threat will eventually lead to better health-related behaviors [10]. By contrast, another study found no correlation between knowledge and behavior [28]. Furthermore, the difference in the proportion of good attitudes with frequent COVID-19 prevention behaviour is also significant, indicating that a good attitude is followed by good behaviour. These results differ slightly from another study conducted in Indonesia. Yanti et al., suggested that Indonesians tend to have good knowledge and a positive attitude, which leads to good behavior [4]. The tendencies are similar to our findings, yet we find no correlation between knowledge and attitude.

However, Yanti et al., only investigated the social distancing policy while we also examined other attitudes and behaviours.

The strengths of the study in this chapter are (1) the large number of respondents covering Sumatera and Java, the most populated islands in Indonesia, which contributed up to 60-70% of COVID-19 cases in Indonesia, and (2) the high internal consistency of the questionnaire. Therefore, this chapter is expected to contribute to controlling COVID-19 in Indonesia through the role of students. However, research with respondents, including students from outside Sumatra and Java islands, is still needed to cover a wider population. This chapter will be used as a database for developing activity programmes to improve students' knowledge, attitude and behaviour for COVID-19 prevention in Indonesia.

Conclusion

Health science students tended to have better knowledge of and better behaviour scores for COVID-19 prevention than those studying in non-health fields. Both knowledge and attitude scores had a significant relationship with behaviour scores, where students with sufficient knowledge and good attitudes were more likely to have good behaviour as well, although no significant relationship was found between knowledge and attitude. Besides student type, gender and household income might also play a significant role. Female students and those with a monthly household income ≥IDR 3,500,000 were more likely to have good attitude and behaviour scores. These findings suggest the need for intervention to optimise the roles of students, both from health and non-health fields and from any sociodemographic and socio-economic background, in contributing to overcoming the rapid spread of COVID-19.

Competing Interests

We declare there is no conflict of interest in this research.

Acknowledgments

We would like to thank our Local Officer on Research Exchange (LORE) and the Center for Indonesian Medical Students' Activities (CIMSA) for their support and help. This article was presented at the 6th International Conference and Exhibition on Indonesian Medical Education and Research Institute (6th ICE on IMERI), Faculty of Medicine, Universitas Indonesia. We thank the 6th ICE on the IMERI committee, who had supported the peer review and manuscript preparation for publication to Nova Science Publishers, Inc.

References

[1] Lotfi M., Hamblin M. R., Rezaei N. COVID-19: transmission, prevention, and potential therapeutic opportunities. *Clin Chim Acta.* 2020 Sep; 508: 254-66.

[2] World Health Organization. *Coronavirus disease (COVID-19) weekly epidemiological update [Internet].* Geneva: World Health Organization; 2021 [Cited 2021 Apr]. Available from: https://www.who.int/publications/m/item/weekly-epidemiological-update-on-covid-19-6-april-2021.

[3] Riyanti D., Jonathan L, Davin S, Aruminingsih S, Mochamad I. Budi H, et al., Review and analysis of current responses to COVID-19 in indonesia: period of january to march 2020. *Progress in Disaster Science*. 2020 Apr; 6: 1000091.

[4] Yanti B., Wahyudi E., Wahiduddin W., Novika R., Arina Y., Martani N., et al., Community knowledge, attitudes, and behavior towards social distancing policy as prevention transmission of COVID-19 in Indonesia. *Jurnal Administrasi Kesehatan Indonesia* [Indonesian Journal of Healthcare Administration]. 2020; 8(2): 4.

[5] Kim J. H., Marks F., Clemens J. D. Looking beyond COVID-19 vaccine phase 3 trials. *Nat Med.* 2021; 27: 205-11.

[6] Husada D. SARS-CoV-2 vaccine: literature review. *J Indones Med Assoc.* 2020; 70(10): 228-42.

[7] Rochanah R. The role of iain kudus pgmi students as agents of change during the COVID-19 pandemic. *Elem Islam Teach J.* 2020; 8(2):339.

[8] Sukaesih, U., Budi S., Sari D. N. Knowledge and attitudes of health students about COVID-19 prevention in indonesia. Jurnal Ilmu Keperawatan dan Kebidanan [*Journal of Nursing and Obstetrics*]. 2020; 11(2): 410-4.

[9] Ernawati K., Cantika I. B., Isaputri R. R., Andari A. W., Ramadhan M. F., Nathasia S. K., et al., Community knowledge, attitudes and behaviors in prevention of COVID-19 transmission: a systematic review. *Int J Public Heal Sci.* 2021; 10(1): 16-26.

[10] Jones C. L., Jensen J. D., Scherr C. L., Brown N. R., Christy K., Weaver J. The health belief model as an explanatory framework in communication research: exploring parallel, serial, and moderated mediation. *Health Commun.* 2015; 30(6): 566-76.

[11] Putra A. I., Pratiwi M. S., Yani M. V., Gunawan G. R., Ganesha G. M., Aminawati A. M., et al., Description of the characteristics of knowledge, attitude and behaviors of COVID-19 risk within traditional village framework in gulingan village, mengwi, bali. J Kesehat Andalas [*Andalas Journal of Health*]. 2020; 9(3): 313-9.

[12] Mujiburrahman, R. M. E., Ningsih M. U. Knowledge is related to increasing COVID-19 prevention behavior in the community. J Keperawatan Terpadu [*Integrated Journal of Nursery*]. 2020; 2(2):130-40.

[13] Mudawaroch R. E. The influence of knowledge and attitudes on student behavior in dealing with the corona virus. *Pros HUBISINTEK.* 2020; 362: 257-63.

[14] Zhong B., Luo W., Li H., Zhang Q., Liu W., Li Y. Knowledge, attitudes, and practices towards COVID-19 among chinese residents during the rapid rise period of the COVID-19 outbreak: a quick online cross-sectional survey. *Int J Biol Sci.* 2020; 16(10): 1745-52.

[15] Olum R., Checkwech G., Wekha G., Nassozi D. R., Bongomin F. Coronavirus disease-2019: knowledge, attitude, and practices of health care workers at makerere university teaching hospitals, uganda. *Front Public Health.* 2020; 8: 181.

[16] Quetionnaire. Survey of community behavior during the pandemic. *Jakarta: Indonesia Central Bureau of Statistics;* 2020 [Cited 2021 Jan]. Available from: https://covid-19.bps.go.id/assets/doc/3-Kuesioner-SurveI-Perilaku-Masy-di-Masa-Pandemi.pdf.

[17] Maheshwari S., Gupta P. K., Sinha R., Rawat P. Knowledge, attitude, and practice towards coronavirus disease 2019 (COVID-19) among medical students: a cross-sectional Study." *J Acute Dis.* 2020; 9(3):100-4.

[18] Alzoubi H., Alnawaiseh N., Al-Mnayyis A., Abu-Lubada M., Aqel Y., Al-Shagahin H. COVID-19 - knowledge, attitude and practice among medical and non-medical university students in jordan. *J Pure Appl Microbiol.* 2020; 14(1): 17-24.

[19] Peng Y., Pei C., Zheng Y. A cross-sectional survey of knowledge, attitude, and practice associated with COVID-19 among undergraduate students in china. *BMC Public Health.* 2021: 1292.

[20] Wonok M. J., Wowor R., Tucunan A. A. Description of community behavior regarding the prevention of COVID-19 in tumani village, maesan district, south minahasa regency. *J KESMAS.* 2020; 9(7): 147-56.

[21] Amarie A., Udijono A., Kusariana N., Saraswati L. D. Description of knowledge, attitude, and practice of coronavirus disease-19 prevention based on gender and age in the java island community. *J Public Heal Trop Coast Reg.* 2020; 3(2):26-30.

[22] Prihati D. R., Wirawati M. K., Supriyanti E. analysis of community knowledge and behavior in kotawaringin barat baru village about COVID-19. *Malahayati Nurs J.* 2020; 2(4): 780-90.

[23] Galasso V., Pons V., Profeta P., Becher M., Brouard S., Foucault M. Gender differences in COVID-19 attitudes and behavior: panel evidence from eight countries. *Proc Natl Acad Sci USA.* 2020; 117(44): 27285-91.

[24] Mujani S., Irvani D. 2020. "Citizen's Attitudes and Behaviors towards Policies for Handling COVID-19 Outbreak." *Polit J Ilmu Polit* 11(2):219-38.

[25] Deeks A., Lombard C., Michelmore J., Teede H. The effects of gender and age on health-related behaviors. *BMC Public Health.* 2009; 9: 1-8.

[26] Moudy J., Sriwijaya U., Syakurah R., Sriwijaya U. Knowledge related toward effort to prevent COVID-19 in indonesia. *J Public Health Res Develop.* 2020; 4(3): 333-46.

[27] Update on the COVID-19 situation in Indonesia, monitoring of health protocol compliance and progress of regional command post. *Jakarta: COVID-19 National Task Force;* 2021 [Cited 2021 Mar]. Available from: https://covid19.go.id/berita/monitoring-kepatuhan-protokol-kesehatan-tingkat-nasional-update-7-maret-2021

[28] Yıldırım M., Güler A. COVID-19 severity, self-efficacy, knowledge, preventive behaviors, and mental health in turkey." *Death Studies*. 2020; 1-8.

Chapter 2

An Analysis of Cardiopulmonary Variables during Exercise While Using Cloth Masks

Mochammad Ridwan[1], Shabrina Narasati[1,*], M. Barlian Nugroho[1], Rahmad[1], Cholid Tri Tjahjono[2], Holipah[3] and Mohammad Saifur Rohman[2]

[1]Department of Physical Medicine and Rehabilitation, Faculty of Medicine, Universitas Brawijaya, Malang, Jawa Timur, Indonesia
[2]Department of Department Cardiology and Vascular Medicine, Faculty of Medicine, Universitas Brawijaya, Malang, Jawa Timur, Indonesia
[3]Department of Public Health, Faculty of Medicine, Universitas Brawijaya, Malang, Jawa Timur, Indonesia

Abstract

Objective: To evaluate the effect of wearing cloth face masks on cardiopulmonary and metabolic physiology and to determine the effect of using a cloth face mask on subjective sensation during low- and moderate-intensity exercise.

Design: We conducted a controlled clinical trial on healthy adults aged between 17 and 35 years. Each subject ran on a treadmill at a speed of 5.6 km/h (low-moderate intensity) for 30 minutes using no mask and then again while wearing a cloth mask. The subjects were then measured for cardiopulmonary and metabolic parameters.

Result: No statistically significant differences were observed in oxygen saturation, respiratory rate, heart rate, blood pressure, end-tidal

* Corresponding Author's Email: shabrina@student.ub.ac.id.

In: The 6th Annual International Conference …
Editors: M. Maidarti, H. Winarto, C. O. M. Jasirwan et al.
ISBN: 978-1-68507-925-3

CO_2 or on the Borg scale. Subjective sensations of humidity, hotness, breath resistance and overall discomfort increases after exercising with a cloth mask.

Conclusion: The use of cloth mask did not cause debilitating physiological and metabolic effects. Subjective sensation of discomfort while wearing a cloth mask is a problem when doing low- and moderate-intensity exercise.

Keywords: personal protective equipment, cloth mask, cardiopulmonary, metabolic, subjective sensations

Introduction

Originating since the 1800s as a way to protect doctors from contracting the miasma, which was thought to be the cause of the bubonic plague, face masks are now used not only in clinical practice but also in public settings [1]. In the era of the Coronavirus Disease 19 (COVID-19), the use of face masks in public places became mandatory in almost every country. COVID-19 is known to be contracted from droplets. Hence, the World Health Organization (WHO) recommended that people use face masks to protect them from inhaling viruses containing droplets from other people. In addition to using masks, the WHO's guidelines also mentioned hand hygiene and social distancing as protective measures against the virus [2, 3]. Therefore, during the COVID-19 pandemic, many people wore cloth face masks rather than surgical or respirator masks.

Many types of masks are now available for different purposes of use. The most common masks are cloth, surgical and respirator masks. However, in general, people do not know the advantages and disadvantages of using cloth face masks on the body's physiology. At the beginning of the COVID-19 pandemic, the demand for surgical face masks outweighed the supply. Hence, the healthcare workers and facilities faced a shortage of masks. Since then, the WHO has recommended that cloth masks be used by the public on a daily basis to reduce surgical mask use and solve the shortage of masks in healthcare facilities [3]. Cloth masks, as the name suggests, are made from cloth material. Cloth face masks can be made from cotton, shirts, sweatshirts or even towels. Compared with surgical and respirator masks, such as N95 masks, face masks made of cloth have the lowest efficiency in filtration, with a filtration efficiency of 2%-40%, depending on the fabric used to make the mask and the layers of fabric used. The denser and more multi-layered the fabric, the higher the filtration efficiency [4]. However, with more dense and layered materials, people often complain about discomfort while wearing cloth face masks. A prior study reported that while using a mask, the wearer experiences difficulty breathing and communicating, increased sweating, and even dermatological issues such as rashes and acne [5]. These complaints raise concerns as they potentially reduce people's compliance with wearing masks.

Many people do not know the effect of wearing a cloth face mask on physical activities with low and moderate intensity. Therefore, this article evaluates the effect of cloth face masks on cardiopulmonary parameters such as oxygen saturation, respiratory rate, heart rate, blood pressure, end-tidal CO_2, talk test, Borg scale and subjective indicators, as well as on metabolic parameters such as blood lactate concentration and body temperature. It is important to understand the effect of cloth face masks, as they are the most common type of face mask used and the most available mask for the public in this COVID-19 pandemic. The results of this chapter can be used by lawmakers when considering face mask regulations for the public.

Materials and Methods

Study Population

This chapter was approved by the board of ethics at Dr Saiful Anwar Hospital, Universitas Brawijaya, Malang, Indonesia. To be included, subjects were required to be healthy adults aged between 17 and 35 years without cardiopulmonary, neuromuscular and musculoskeletal disorders, and with a body mass index (BMI) of 18.5-24.99 kg/m^2. Before study initiation, signed informed consent was obtained from all participants. Pregnant participants were excluded. Participants who did not complete the research protocol and had to be terminated while performing the tests were categorised as dropouts. The absolute indications for test termination were as follows: (a) participant's request, (b) acute myocardial infarction, (c) moderate-severe angina pectoris, (d) ST segment elevation $\geq$1 mm in leads without pathological Q waves, (e) systolic pressure drops >10 mmHg below systolic pressure at rest while standing with evidence of ischemia, or >20 mmHg after a previous systolic increase, (f) severe arrhythmias (AV Block degree 2 or 3, VT or VF) and

(g) technical problems. The relative indications for termination were as follows: (a) depression in the ST segment >2 mm, (b) severe chest pain, (c) tightness, fatigue, leg cramps or claudication, (d) systolic blood pressure ≥230 mmHg, diastolic ≥115 mmHg, (e) systolic pressure drops >10 mmHg below systolic pressure at rest standing with evidence of ischemia, (f) arrhythmias (PVC, SVT, bradyarrhythmia, grade 1 AV block) that can potentially disturb hemodynamics and (g) bundle branch block. Sampling was carried out using consecutive sampling. Participants who fit the study criteria were included in the study.

Data Collection and Outcome

Each subject ran on a treadmill at a 5.6 km/h speed (low-moderate intensity) for 30 minutes. The procedure consisted of a warm-up, exercise and rest. The subject underwent the procedure twice, first without a mask and then while wearing a cloth mask. The patients were then instructed to cool down by walking until their heart rate dropped below 100 beats per minute. All the participants wore athletic clothing and shoes. Figure 1 shows the timing of the metabolic and physiological parameter measurements. The subjects were wearing a Withleof® handheld pulse oximeter and capnograph to monitor oxygen saturation, heart rate and End-tidal CO_2. The Borg rating of perceived exertion (Borg scale) was used to measure the physical sensations experienced by the subjects. The scale starts from 6, indicating no exertion at all, to 20, indicating maximal exertion. Blood lactate was measured using capillary blood, which was then inserted into Accutrend® Plus Lactate. Blood glucose was also measured using capillary blood and inserted into Accutrend® Plus Glucose. The talk test was conducted according to previous studies [6, 7]. The participants joined in a conversation with the examiner, and the examiner determined how the subject talked. For the statistical analysis, the intensity of the exercise - light, moderate and vigorous - were represented by 1, 2 and 3, respectively. Body temperature was measured using an infrared thermometer. All participants were given a form that contained a subjective sensations scale and were asked to rate each sensation from 0 (not at all) to 10 (strongly) before exercising and again after they finished exercising. The subjective sensation scale was adopted from a previous study by Li et al. [8].

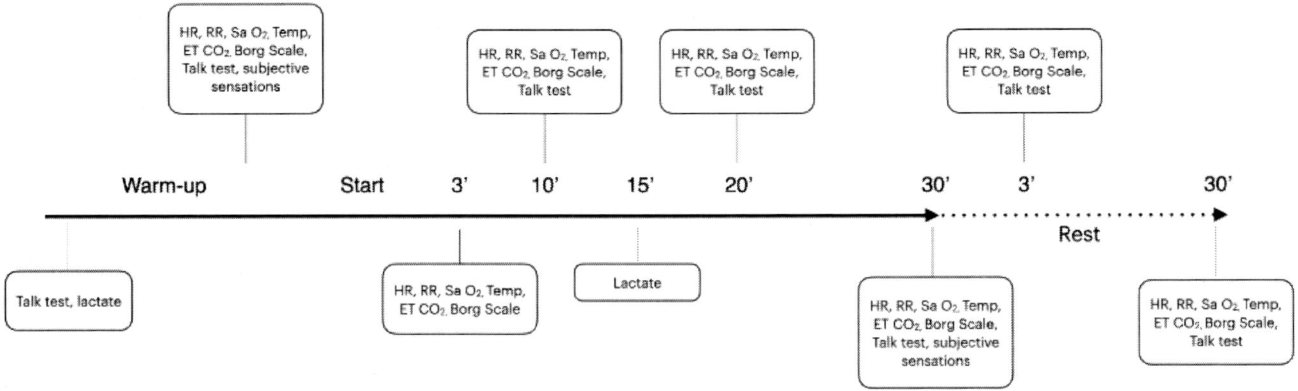

(HR = heart rate, RR = respiratory rate, Sa O_2 = Oxygen saturation, Temp = body temperature, ET CO_2 = end-tidal CO_2).

Figure 1. Physiological and metabolic parameters' measurement.

Statistical Analysis

The master table was used to record data that were gathered in this chapter. SPSS version 23.0 and GraphPad version 9.1.0 were used to analyse the data. The Shapiro-Wilke's test was used to determine the normality of numerical data, after which homogeneous or normally distributed data ($p > .05$) were presented with mean and standard deviation (SD), while data that were not normally distributed ($p > .05$) were presented with the median (minimum value; maximum value). Pairwise comparison using the 2-way ANOVA non-parametric test was used to examine the relationship between variables with non-homogeneous results. A statistically significant correlation is shown by a p-value less than .005 (95% significance). If a significant value was obtained, a post-hoc multiple comparison analysis was performed using Dunn's test. The relationship between the ordinal data was analysed using a non-parametric pairwise comparative with Friedman's 2-way ANOVA test. A p-value below 0.05 indicates a statistically significant correlation (95% significance). If a significant value was obtained, a post hoc pair-wise comparison analysis was performed using Bonferroni's correction.

Results

Subjects' Characteristics

Ten participants were recruited in this chapter, comprising five males and five females. Baseline characteristics (Table 1), including gender, age, weight, height and BMI, were recorded. Participant's ages ranged from 22 to 29 years old, mean weight was 55.90 ± 11.32 kilograms, mean height was 162.8 ± 8.2 cm and mean BMI was 20.97 ± 3.0 kg/m^2. No statistical significance difference was found in the baseline characteristics.

Table 1. Baseline Characteristics

Characteristics	Mean ± SD	p-value
Age (years)	25.10 ± 2.2	.064
Weight (kg)	55.90 ± 11.32	.571
Height (cm)	162.8 ± 8.2	.506
BMI (kg/m^2)	20.97 ± 3.0	.995

* statistically significant (p-value < .05).

Physiologic and Metabolic Parameters

Table 2 reports the median, minimum and maximum values of respiratory rate, heart rate, oxygen saturation, end-tidal CO_2, body temperature, Borg scale, blood lactate and talk test in the control and cloth mask groups. A comparison of the two groups resulted in no statistically significant difference in all aforementioned parameters, except for the talk test ($p = .0054$). Table 3 reports the median, minimum and maximum values for subjective sensation while using a cloth mask. For the sensation of humid, hot, breath resistance and overall discomfort, a statistical significance was found between before and after the exercise.

Discussion

Face masks were created as a barrier between the outside environment and our upper airways to reduce the risk of inhaling infectious agents or dangerous chemicals and particles. Because the face mask acts as a barrier, it causes resistance to airflow. Hence, it is useful to identify whether the use of a face mask impacts our physiological functions. The COVID-19 pandemic situation obliged almost everyone in every country to use masks to reduce virus transmission. Several issues have then arisen regarding the discomfort felt while using face masks.

A previous study of 402 subjects reported that as much as 78.4% of the respondents reported discomfort while wearing a face mask [5]. This issue caused non-compliance with wearing face masks and increased the level of anxiety felt by the wearer [5, 9]. This reaction to face masks has become a problem as the number of people infected with COVID-19 is still increasing.

Our data indicate that the use of cloth masks did not alter physiological functions such as respiratory rate, heart rate, oxygen saturation, end-tidal CO_2, body temperature and blood lactate in low-to-moderate-intensity workload or exercise. In accordance with our study, previous research has also reported similar results that showed the use of face masks did not alter gas exchange, ventilation or thermoregulation [10, 11]. However, when using cloth masks, participants tend to have difficulty talking and have increased sensations of humidity, hotness, breathing resistance and discomfort in general. A similar result was also reported by Li et al., [8] who compared the effect of wearing an N95 respirator mask with a surgical mask on subjective sensations. This

Table 2. Physiologic and metabolic parameters before, during, and after exercise

Mask	0 min	After warm-up	3 min	10 min	15 min	20 min	30 min	3 min rest	30 min rest
Respiratory rate (breath/min)									
Control	16 (12;20)	-	21 (12;30)	26.5 (13;33)	-	27.5 (18;44)	26 (18;40)	20.5 (12;33)	16 (12;27)
Cloth mask	19 (13;24)	-	21 (14;32)	26.5 (16;32)	-	27 (15;35)	24.5 (17;35)	23 (13;32)	16 (12;27)
Heart rate (bpm)									
Control	87 (77;112)	-	107.5 (82;128)	135 (102;174)	-	136 (109;170)	140 (108;167)	118.5 (86;140)	100 (79;123)
Cloth mask	95 (82;110)	-	110 (89;150)	127 (107;170)	-	141 (108;155)	127 (107;151)	117 (102;141)	98.5 (79;119)
Oxygen saturation (%)									
Control	98 (98;99)	-	98 (96;99)	96.5 (94;99)	-	98 (96;99)	97 (96;98)	97 (97;98)	97.5 (96;99)
Cloth mask	97 (96;99)	-	97.5 (96;99)	97 (96;98)	-	97.5 (96;98)	97 (95;99)	97 (97;99)	97.5 (96;99)
End-tidal CO_2 (%)									
Control	34 (29;38)	-	38 (35;50)	40 (32;46)	-	37.5 (29;48)	39 (27;49)	35.5 (26;40)	31.5 (27;39)
Cloth mask	37.5 (32;39)	-	41 (38;47)	43.5 (38;48)	-	43 (35;48)	41.5 (36;48)	37 (32;44)	35.5 (32;40)
Body temperature (°C)									
Control	36.4 (36.3;36.9)	-	36.4 (36.2;36.9)	36.4 (36.1;36.8)	-	36.3 (36.1;36.7)	36.35 (36;36.6)	36.3 (35.5;36.8)	36.4 (36;36.7)
Cloth mask	36.4 (36.3;36.6)	-	36.4 (36;36.6)	36.3 (35.6;36.6)	-	36.3 (36.1;36.8)	36.3 (36.1;36.8)	36.3 (36;36.8)	36.4 (36.1;36.7)
Borg scale									
Control	6 (6;7)	-	7 (6;12)	12 (6;14)	-	14 (8;15)	15 (8;15)	9 (6;14)	6 (6;7)
Cloth mask	6 (6;7)	-	6 (6;11)	8 (8;13)	-	10 (8;15)	11 (8;15)	7.5 (6;11)	6 (6;11)
Blood lactate (mmol/L)									
Control	1.65 (0.9;2.7)	-		-	4.2 (1.6;10.4)	-	-	4 (1.9;10.6)	2.1 (1.0;5.2)
Cloth mask	2.1 (0.9;5.4)	-		-	4.2 (1.9;6.8)	-	-	3.4 (1.8;5.8)	1.9 (1.6;3.3)
Talk test									
Control	1 (1;1)	1 (1;1)		1 (1;2)	-	2 (1;2)	2 (1;2)	1 (1;1)	1 (1;1)
Cloth mask*	1 (1;1)	1 (1;1)		1 (1;1)	-	1 (1;1)	1 (1;2)	1 (1;1)	1 (1;1)

Note: Values are median (minimum;maximum). * statistically significant in main effect comparison (p-value < .05).

Table 3. Subjective sensations measurement while wearing a cloth mask

Subjective sensations		**Humid**	**Hot**	**Breath Resistance**	**Itchy**	**Tight**	**Salty**	**Unfit**	**Odour**	**Fatigue**	**Overall Discomfort**
Cloth mask	Before	0 (0;3)	1 (0;2)	0 (0;4)	0 (0;1)	0 (0;5)	0 (0;1)	0 (0;1)	0 (0;3)	0 (0;2)	1 (0;2)
	After	4.5 (0;7)	4.5 (2;6)	2 (0;4)	0 (0;2)	0.5 (0;5)	0 (0;1)	0 (0;1)	0.5 (0;3)	0 (0;5)	2.5 (0;4)
	p-value	<0.001*	<0.001*	0.023*	0.660	0.423	1	1	0.661	0.224	0.019*

Note: Values are median (minimum;maximum). *statistically significant (p-value $< .05$).

chapter reported a higher discomfort level in the N95 respirator mask as it causes more breathing resistance and tightness on the face. A previous study also suggested that the skin surface on the facial area is more thermosensitive than other parts of the body [12]. Hence, the slightest change in facial skin microenvironment might be perceived more strongly.

In this chapter, we conducted a low- to moderate-intensity workload to replicate the intensity of usual daily activities, and we only tested the use of a cloth mask for 30 minutes. A previous study reported that most mask wearers use it for 4-6 hours daily [5]. Hence, the results of physiological and metabolic parameters might be different with longer usage times. Different intensity of exercise or activities might also produce different results. Driver et al. [13] determined the physiological effect of cloth masks in low-, moderate- and high-intensity exercise. A statistically significant difference was reported in oxygen saturation and heart rate during high-intensity exercise. Hence, special considerations should be made towards people who exercise using face masks.

Besides the evidence provided, this chapter has several limitations. The method to measure cardiopulmonary parameters is not a gold standard method. We also cannot exclude the subjectivity of the patient in the assessment of subjective sensation.

Conclusion

There is no effect on the physiological or metabolic rate of the healthy subjects who use cloth masks. However, the discomfort sensation while wearing the masks is the biggest concern during low- to moderate-intensity exercise.

Acknowledgments

This article was presented at the 6th International Conference and Exhibition on Indonesian Medical Education and Research Institute (6th ICE on IMERI), Faculty of Medicine, Universitas Indonesia. We thank the 6th ICE on the IMERI committee, who had supported the peer review and manuscript preparation for publication to Nova Science Publishers, Inc.

Competing Interests: The authors declare no conflicts of interest.

References

[1] Matuschek C, Moll F, Fangerau H, Fischer JC, Zanker K, van Griensven M. The history and value of face masks. *Eur. J. Med. Res.* 2020; 25: 23.

[2] World Health Organization. Mask use in the context of COVID-19 [Internet]. Geneva: World Health Organization; 2020 [Cited 2021 May]. Available from: https://apps.who.int/iris/bitstream/handle/10665/337199/WHO-2019-nCov-IPC_Masks-2020.5-eng.pdf?sequence=1&isAllowed=y.

[3] World Health Organization. When and how to use masks [Internet]. Geneva: World Health Organization; 2021 [Cited 2021 May]. Available from: https://www.who.int/emergencies/diseases/novel-coronavirus-2019/advice-for-public/when-and-how-to-use-masks.

[4] Sharma S, Mishra M, Mudgal S. Efficacy of cloth face mask in prevention of novel coronavirus infection transmission: a systematic review and meta-analysis. *J. Educ. Health Promot*. 2020; 9: 192.

[5] Cheok GJ, Gatot C, Sim CH, Ng YH, Tay KX, Howe TS, et al. Appropriate attitude promotes mask wearing in spite of a significant experience of varying discomfort. *Infect. Dis. Heal.* 2021; 26(2):145-51.

[6] Reed JL, Pipe AL. The talk test: a useful tool for prescribing and monitoring exercise intensity. *Curr. Opin. Cardiol*. 2014: 29.

[7] Reed JL, Pipe AL. Practical approaches to prescribing physical activity and monitoring exercise intensity. *Can. J. Cardiol*. 2016; 32(4): 514-22.

[8] Li Y, Tokura H, Guo YP, Wong AS, Wong T, Chung J, et al. Effects of wearing N95 and surgical facemasks on heart rate, thermal stress and subjective sensations. *Int. Arch. Occup. Environ. Health*. 2005; 78(6): 501-9.

[9] Wu S, Harber P, Yun D, Bansal S, Li Y, Santiago S. Anxiety during respirator use: comparison of two respirator types. *J. Occup. Environ. Hyg*. 2011; 8(3): 123-8.

[10] Haraf RH, Faghy MA, Carlin B, Josephson RA. The physiological impact of masking is insignificant and should not preclude routine use during daily activities, exercise, and rehabilitation. *J. Cardiopulm. Rehabil. Prev*. 2021; 41(1): 1-5.

[11] Shein SL, Whitticar S, Mascho KK, Pace E, Speicher R, Deakins K. The effects of wearing facemasks on oxygenation and ventilation at rest and during physical activity. *PLoS One*. 2021; 16(2): e0247414.

[12] Roberge RJ, Kim JH, Coca A. Protective facemask impact on human thermoregulation: an overview. *Ann. Occup. Hyg*. 2012; 56:102-12.

[13] Driver S, Reynolds M, Brown K, Vingren JL, Hill DW, Bennett M, et al. Effects of wearing a cloth face mask on performance, physiological and perceptual responses during a graded treadmill running exercise test. *Br. J. Sports Med*. 2021: 1-7.

Chapter 3

Analysis of FoxM1 Expression in Sinonasal Inverted Papilloma and Sinonasal Inverted Papilloma with Dysplastic Changes

Lisnawati Rachmadi*, **Yayi Dwina and David Sitinjak**
Anatomical Pathology Department, Faculty of Medicine, Universitas Indonesia – Dr Cipto Mangunkusumo General Hospital, Jakarta, Indonesia

Abstract

Sinonasal papilloma is an uncommon benign neoplasm arising from sinonasal surface epithelia. Sinonasal papilloma has a propensity to undergo malignant transformation. A new biomarker recently reported being involved in malignant transformation in sinonasal papilloma to be sinonasal squamous cell carcinoma. FoxM1 is a transcription factor whose primary role in carcinogenesis is in cellular proliferation and cell cycle regulation.

Purpose: This study describes the expression of FoxM1 in sinonasal inverted papilloma and its association with dysplastic changes.

Methods: A cross-sectional, analytical study comprised 36 histologically confirmed diagnoses of inverted papilloma slides between 2014 and 2019. The samples were further grouped into 21 samples without associated dysplastic changes and 15 samples with associated dysplastic changes. FoxM1 immunostaining was performed in all samples, and the percentage of positively stained cells was compared among the two groups using appropriate comparative statistics.

Results: The mean percentage of positively stained cells in inverted papilloma without associated dysplastic changes is 7.4% (SD±1.67), and

* Corresponding Author's Email: lisnawatidr@gmail.com.

In: The 6th Annual International Conference …
Editors: M. Maidarti, H. Winarto, C. O. M. Jasirwan et al.
ISBN: 978-1-68507-925-3

with associated dysplastic changes it is 33.5% (SD±14.77). A statistically significant difference was evident in FoxM1 expression between the two groups ($p < .001$). Expression of FoxM1 was found to be higher in the inverted papilloma with associated dysplastic changes.

Conclusion: FoxM1 immunostaining has the potential to be a biomarker of malignant transformation in sinonasal inverted papilloma.

Keywords: inverted papilloma, FoxM1, dysplasia

Introduction

Sinonasal papilloma is a benign growth of surface epithelia (the pseudo-stratified ciliated or Schneiderian epithelia) that line the nasal cavity and sinonasal tract. Sinonasal papilloma is uncommon: collectively, they comprise only about 4% of all sinonasal neoplasms [1]. Inverted sinonasal papilloma (ISP) is one type of sinonasal papilloma characterised by its inward epithelial growth towards stroma. Compared to other histological types (oncocytic and exophytic), about 5-15% of inverted papilloma tends to recur and undergo a malignant transformation [2].

The mechanism of malignant transformation in sinonasal papilloma has not been fully understood. Inflammation, the imbalance between cell proliferation and apoptosis, and adhesion molecule involvement are assumed to play a role in the malignant transformation of ISP [3]. The role of Human papillomavirus (HPV) in ISP remains contradictory [2]. Recent studies have found a critical molecular alteration in sinonasal papilloma. Epidermal growth factor receptor (EGFR) mutations are found in 88% of cases of inverted papilloma [4]. Numerous molecules, including FoxM1, have recently been reported to be overexpressed in the malignant transformation of ISP [5]. FoxM1 is a transcription factor belonging to the Forkhead family. Its transcriptional regulator function is linked to the carcinogenesis process towards cellular proliferation regulation and cell cycle progression [6]. Moreover, in human epithelial cancers, FoxM1 is correlated with tumour initiation, progression and metastasis [7].

This chapter evaluates FoxM1 expression in a series of ISP with/without dysplasia and compares the proportion of positively stained epithelial cells among groups: ISP without dysplasia, ISP with low- to moderate-grade dysplasia and ISP with high-grade dysplasia.

Materials and Methods

We conducted a single-centre retrospective cohort study of consecutive patients histologically diagnosed with ISP in our institution from January 2014 to December 2019. The study was conducted after obtaining ethical approval from the Ethics Committee of the Faculty of Medicine Universitas Indonesia. Inclusion criteria were patients with evidence of sinonasal papilloma on histopathology, who underwent surgical procedures at Dr Cipto Mangunkusumo General Hospital (CMH), and with accessible histologic slides and paraffin blocks from the tissue archive, Department of Anatomical Pathology, Dr Cipto Mangunkusumo General Hospital, Jakarta, Indonesia. We used minimal sample size calculation using the formula for an unpaired comparative study. The mean difference used in the formula is based on a previous study by Wang et al. [5]. Based on the calculation, the minimal sample size per group was 15. The patient's demographics, symptoms, type of surgery, recurrence, malignant transformation and radiological data were reviewed retrospectively using the patient's medical records. Krouse staging was used according to radiographic information. The authors examined the histopathologic specimens retrospectively, based on hematoxylin- and eosin-stained slides. All slides are recorded for histologic grade. Previous studies used modified histological grading systems [8].

IHC Staining

Sections of formalin-fixed, paraffin-embedded tissues were prepared for immunohistochemical analysis. Following deparaffinisation and rehydration, the specimens were incubated with rabbit monoclonal anti-FoxM1 (EPR17379; Abcam, Cambridge, UK) at a dilution of 1:250, then incubated with the anti-rabbit peroxidase-conjugated secondary antibody (Novolink, Illinois, USA) for 30 minutes. Diaminobenzidine was used as a chromogen, and the sections were counterstained with hematoxylin and coverslipped. Two authors (pathologists) performed a separate and blinded review of the immunohistochemistry slides. FoxM1 is localised in the nucleus. Therefore, FoxM1 was assessed quantitatively as the percentage of cells with positive staining in 10 random high power fields. To minimise the subjective aspect of quantification, we used QuPath v0.2.3, image analysis software, to count the 'positive' cells and 'negative' cells automatically.

Statistical Analysis

All data were analysed using SPSS software version 20.0 (SPSS Inc., Chicago, IL). Statistical analysis was performed using ANOVA followed by the Tamhane post hoc test. A p-value of .05 was used as the threshold for statistical significance.

Results

Patient Characteristics

Based on the records of 36 patients with a histologically confirmed diagnosis of ISP either without dysplasia (N = 21 patients) or with dysplasia (N = 15 patients), tissues from 26 men and 10 women were retrospectively reviewed and enrolled in this study. Demographic and clinical data (sex, patient's age, chief complaint, type of surgery, and recurrence) were collected and are presented in Table 1.

Table 1. Patients' clinical characteristics

Variables	ISP				Total (n = 36)		Note
	Without Dysplasia (n = 21)		With Dysplasia (n = 15)				
Age (in years; mean, SD)	53 ± 11,8		49 ± 9,3		51 ± 10,8		***P*** = .293[a]
Sex							
Male	15	(71%)	1	(73%)	26	(72%)	***P*** = .900[b]
Female	6	(29%)	1	(27%)	10	(28%)	
			4				
Chief complaint							
Nasal congestion	14	(67%)	5	(33%)	19	(53%)	n/a
Epistaxis	2	(10%)	1	(7%)	3	(8%)	
Facial mass	1	(5%)	2	(13%)	3	(8%)	
Facial pain	0	0	1	(7%)	1	(3%)	
Rhinorrhoea	1	(5%)	0	0	1	(3%)	
Other symptoms	2	(10%)	2	(13%)	4	(11%)	
No data	1	(5%)	4	(27%)	5	(14%)	
Surgery							
Functional endoscopic sinus	17	(81%)	5	(33%)	22	(61%)	n/a
surgery (FESS)	4	(19%)	9	(60%)	13	(36%)	
Open resection	0	0	1	(7%)	1	(3%)	

Variables	ISP				Total (n = 36)		Note
	Without Dysplasia (n = 21)		With Dysplasia (n = 15)				
Biopsy per nasoendoscopy							
Recurrence							
Single	3	(14%)	3	(20%)	6	(17%)	n/a
Multiple	0	0	5	(33%)	5	(14%)	
No recurrence	18	(86%)	7	(47%)	25	(69%)	
Progression toward carcinoma							
Synchronous	0	0	9	(60%)	9	(25%)	n/a
Metachronous	0	0	4	(27%)	4	(11%)	
No progression	21	(100%)	2	(13%)	23	(64%)	

[an] unpaired student t-test
[b] Chi-square test
SD = standard deviation

FoxM1 Expression

From immunohistochemistry staining, FoxM1 expression was observed only in the nuclei of positive cells. In the ISP samples, positive cells were observed mainly in the basal and parabasal layers of hyperplastic epithelia. In the dysplastic component of the ISP samples, the positive cells spread diffusely, approaching the surface of epithelia (Figure 1). The percentage of FoxM1 immunopositivity was found to increase significantly in ISP with malignant transformation ($p < .001$) (Table 2). We also found that the immunopositivity of FoxM1 gradually increased in proportion to the histological grade of ISP with malignant transformation, although it was not supported by statistical calculations. Based on these findings, we can infer that FoxM1 plays a significant role in the malignant transformation of ISP.

Table 2. FoxM1 Expression

Sinonasal inverted papilloma	N	FoxM1 expression (in percentage) mean ± SD	*p*-value
Without dysplasia	21	7,4 ± 1,67	< .001[a]
With dysplasia (combined)	15	33,5 ± 14,77	
Low to moderate-grade	6	24,8 ± 11,70	
High grade	9	39,3 ± 14,22	

[a] one way ANOVA test.

Table 3. Post-Hoc analysis for comparison of FoxM1 expression between groups

Groups	Mean difference	Confidence interval 95%		*P*-values
		Minimum	Maximum	
Without dysplasia vs low to moderate-grade dysplasia	17.4	0.6	34.2	.043*
Without dysplasia vs high grade dysplasia	31.9	17.6	46.1	< .001*
Low to moderate-grade dysplasia vs high-grade dysplasia	14.4	- 4.1	33.0	.149

[a] post hoc Tamhane's test.

* statistically significant.

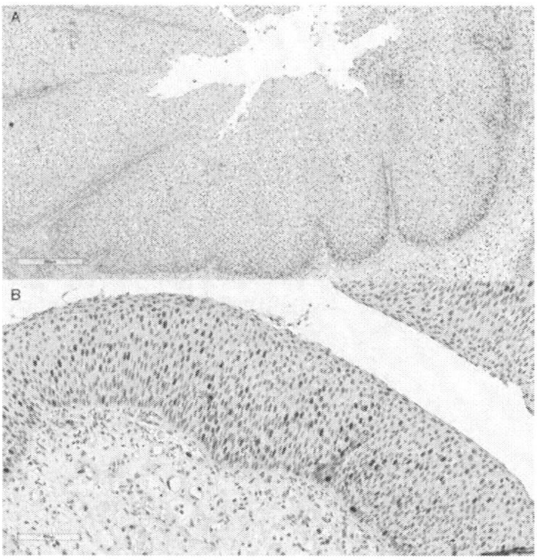

Figure 1. FoxM1 expression in sinonasal inverted papilloma. A. SIP without dysplasia, 10x B. SIP with dysplasia, 20x. FoxM1 immunostaining.

Discussion

ISP is an uncommon benign sinonasal tumour that harbours a tendency towards malignant transformation. Currently, there are no histologic criteria to establish malignant transformation in ISP [9]. The current study explored the role of FoxM1 in the pathophysiology of malignant transformation of ISP.

A previous study conducted by Wang et al., showed the promising role of FoxM1 as a marker of malignant transformation of ISP [5].

This study was conducted using the immunohistochemistry method to visualise the expression and distribution of FoxM1 protein. FoxM1 is a transcription factor that is involved in cellular proliferation. The standard control of FoxM1 expression is increased by proto-oncoprotein (such as c-Myc, AKT, Ras, EGFR, Her-2/neu) and suppressed by tumour suppressor genes (such as Rb, PTEN, p53, GATA3, FoxO3a).10 Because of its role in cellular proliferation, FoxM1 also plays an essential role in carcinogenesis. The amplification of the 12p13 chromosome (the FoxM1 coding gene) is found in several malignancies, i.e., cervical squamous cell carcinoma, breast carcinoma, nasopharyngeal carcinoma and squamous cell carcinoma of the head and neck.6 Moreover, there have been reports on the crosstalk between oncogenic signalling pathways with FoxM1, including the Hedgehog signalling pathway that has been found to upregulate FoxM1 [11].

In squamous cell carcinoma, FoxM1 plays a role in many stages of carcinogenesis, including initiation, progression and metastasis. FoxM1 is upregulated during tumour development in synergy with other carcinogens to produce the premalignant hyperplastic phenotype. It may induce genomic instability, thus starting a series of malignant transformations through epigenetic modifications and genomic instability [12]. FoxM1 is also reported to be upregulated in the malignant transformation of pulmonary adenoma to mucinous adenocarcinoma through activation of the AGR2 gene, the key regulator of a mucinous phenotype [13]. Angiogenesis, an essential phenomenon in carcinogenesis, is also observed in the malignant transformation of ISP. The overexpression of vascular endothelial growth factor (VEGF) increases the number of micro vessels per unit area (MVNA) in ISP. FoxM1 is reported to be involved in the regulation of VEGF [14].

In this study, FoxM1 was overexpressed in the malignant transformation of ISP. We also observed that the increase in FoxM1 corresponded to the histologic degree of malignant transformation. Such a finding helps us understand the molecular pathways of malignant transformation of ISP and will help develop biomarkers for the early detection of malignant transformation in ISP human cancers in general and enrich the available therapeutic approach. ISP is currently treated by complete surgical excision, although recurrences are still reported in 20-30% of cases. Therefore, the positive expression of FoxM1 in ISP could help direct the therapeutic strategy towards targeting FoxM1. However, it should be emphasised that there were several limitations in the study. The sample size was relatively small, even though we used all samples that met the inclusion criteria. Furthermore, the lack of a number in each group of histological degree must be approached cautiously.

Conclusion

In conclusion, this study demonstrated that the expression level of FoxM1 in ISP with dysplasia is significantly higher than in ISP without dysplasia. The expression of FoxM1 was also observed to gradually increase among low-to-moderate grade dysplasia and high-grade dysplasia, although the difference was not statistically significant. We believe the study results provide a basis for investigating the role and function of FoxM1 in ISP and provide a therapeutic target for future clinical management.

Competing Interests

No potential competing interest is disclosed in this study.

Acknowledgments

This article was presented at the 6th International Conference and Exhibition on Indonesian Medical Education and Research Institute (6th ICE on IMERI), Faculty of Medicine, Universitas Indonesia. We thank the 6th ICE on the IMERI committee, who had supported the peer review and manuscript preparation for publication to Nova Science Publishers, Inc.

References

[1] Barnes L. Schneiderian papillomas and nonsalivary glandular neoplasms of the head and neck. *Mod. Pathol.* 2002 Mar; 15(3): 279-97.

[2] Bishop J A. 2017. OSPs and ESPs and ISPs, oh my! an update on sinonasal (schneiderian) papillomas. *Head Neck Pathol*. 2017 Sep; 11(3): 269-77.

[3] Yoon B N, Chon K M, Hong S L, Lee J H, Kim J Y, Cho K S, et al. Inflammation and apoptosis in malignant transformation of sinonasal inverted papilloma: the role

of the bridge molecules, cyclooxygenase-2, and nuclear factor κB. *Am. J. Otolaryngol.* 2013 Feb; 34(1): 22–30.

[4] Udager A M, Rolland D C, McHugh J B, Betz B L, Murga-Zamalloa C, Carey T E, et al. High-frequency targetable EGFR mutations in sinonasal squamous cell carcinomas arising from inverted sinonasal papilloma. *Cancer Res.* 2015 Jul 1; 75(13): 2600-6.

[5] Wang H, Li H, Hu L, Wang J, Liu Q, Wang D, et al. Overexpression of FoxM1 in sinonasal inverted papilloma and associated squamous cell carcinoma. *Am. J. Rhinol. Allergy. 2019* Nov; 33(6): 706-15.

[6] Laoukili J, Stahl M, Medema RH. FoxM1: at the crossroads of ageing and cancer. Biochim Biophys Acta. 2007 Jan; 1775(1): 92-102.

[7] Teh M T. FOXM1 coming of age: time for translation into clinical benefits. *Front Oncol.* 2012; 2: 146.

[8] Roh H J, Procop G W, Batra P S, Citardi M J, Lanza D C. Inflammation and the pathogenesis of inverted papilloma. *Am. J. Rhinol.* Mar-Apr 2004; 18(2): 65-74.

[9] Nudell J, Chiosea S, Thompson L D. Carcinoma ex-schneiderian papilloma (malignant transformation): a clinicopathologic and immunophenotypic study of 20 cases combined with a comprehensive review of the literature. *Head Neck Pathol.* 2014; 8(3): 269-86.

[10] Wierstra I. FOXM1 (forkhead box M1) in tumorigenesis: overexpression in human cancer, implication in tumorigenesis, oncogenic functions, tumor-suppressive properties, and target of anticancer therapy. *Adv. Cancer Res.* 2013; 119: 191-419.

[11] Jaiswal N, Chakraborty S, Nag A. Biology of FOXM1 and its emerging role in cancer therapy. *J. Proteins Proteom.* 2014; 5(1): 1-24.

[12] Gemenetzidis E, Bose A, Riaz A M, Chaplin T, Young B D, Ali M. FOXM1 upregulation is an early event in human squamous cell carcinoma and it is enhanced by nicotine during malignant transformation. *PLoS One*. 2009; 4(3): e4849.

[13] Milewski D, Balli D, Usyiyan V, Le T, Dienemann H. Warth A, et al. FOXM1 activates agr2 and causes progression of lung adenomas into invasive mucinous adenocarcinomas. *PLoS Genet.* 2017 Dec 21; 13(12): e1007097.

[14] Yu H, Liu Q, Wang H, Wang D, Hu L, Sun X, et al. The role of tissue factor pathway inhibitor-2 in malignant transformation of sinonasal inverted papilloma. *Eur. Arch. Otorhinolaryngol.* 2014 Aug; 271(8): 2191-6.

Chapter 4

Comparing the Graded Repetitive Arm Supplementary Program (Grasp) Exercise and Modified Constraint-Induced Movement Therapy (Mcimt) on the Upper Limb Function of Ischemic Stroke Patients: A Randomized Controlled Trial

Herry Hong[1,*], Widjajalaksmi Kusumaningsih[1], Mohammad Kurniawan[2] and Dewi Friska[3]

[1]Department of Medical Rehabilitation, Faculty of Medicine, University of Indonesia, Jakarta, Indonesia
[2]Department of Neurology, Faculty of Medicine, University of Indonesia, Jakarta, Indonesia
[3]Department of Community Medicine, Faculty of Medicine, University of Indonesia, Jakarta, Indonesia

Abstract

Introduction: Upper limb function after stroke is essential for independence in daily activities, and it contributes to the health-related quality of life. *Purpose:* The purpose of this study was to compare the effect of the Graded Repetitive Arm Supplementary Program (GRASP) exercise and modified Constraint-Induced Movement Therapy (mCIMT) on upper limb function in subacute phase ischemic stroke patients. *Methods:* This randomized controlled trial recruited subacute phase first-attack ischemic stroke patients with one-sided hemiparesis. A total of 18

* Corresponding Author's Email: herrymd@gmail.com.

In: The 6th Annual International Conference …
Editors: M. Maidarti, H. Winarto, C. O. M. Jasirwan et al.
ISBN: 978-1-68507-925-3

subjects were divided equally into two exercise groups: the GRASP group (GG) and mCIMT group (CG). The exercise was performed at home for 4 weeks. Then, the upper limb function was assessed using the Fugl-Meyer Assessment Upper Extremity (FMA-UE) and Chedoke Arm and Hand Activity Inventory (CAHAI-13). *Results:* No significant differences were found between the two groups after 2 weeks of training (T1). The FMA-UE mean difference (MD) was 3.67 ± 1.94 in the GG and 3.11 ± 1.54 in the CG ($p = 0.510$). The CAHAI MD was 5.33 ± 3.46 in the GG and 3.11 ± 1.27 in the CG ($p = 0.050$). After 4 weeks of training (T2), no significant differences were found between the two groups; the FMA-UE MD was 8.67 ± 4.47 and 8.56 ± 2.07 ($p = 0.489$) in the GG and CG, respectively, while the CAHAI MD was 13.44 ± 4.85 and 10.11 ± 2.62 ($p = 0.088$) in the GG and CG, respectively. *Conclusions:* It was concluded that GRASP exercise was as effective as mCIMT at improving upper limb function in subacute ischemic stroke patients.

Keywords: upper limb, stroke, exercise therapy

Introduction

Stroke is still the main cause of death and disability in developing countries [1]. The prevalence of stroke in Indonesia increased from 7% in 2013 to 10.9% in 2018. It was predicted that 3.4 million people over 18 years of age will suffer a stroke in Indonesia [2].

Ischemic stroke is the most common type of stroke, representing nearly 80% of all strokes [3]. Ischemic damage induces substantial change to the entire neural system within the involved area, and in response to this damage, the cerebral cortex exhibits some form of spontaneous brain plasticity. These neuroplasticity phenomena are usually found in the perilesional area of the involved hemisphere, but they may also be found in other areas, such as the contralateral hemisphere and subcortical and spinal regions [4].

A stroke patient can recover from his/her condition via reduction in impairment or compensation. The cause of this recovery is multifactorial. In the first 1 to 3 months post-stroke, functional recovery is usually the result of spontaneous reorganization. Patients also achieve increased responsiveness when subjected to enriched environments and/or training. This is attributable to a short-lived sensitive period of post-ischemic plasticity, which is influenced by unique genetic, molecular, physiological, and structural events. In contrast, the process of compensation can occur at any time after stroke [5].

Despite brain plasticity phenomena, approximately 75% of stroke survivors are left with long-lasting motor dysfunction. Although improvements are expected after rehabilitation programmes, approximately 30 to 60% of these patients will be left with persistent impairment of their upper limb function [6-8]. Because of the physiological process of post-ischemic plasticity, early admission to stroke units that include rehabilitation programmes is strongly associated with improved functional recovery.

In a developing country with an archipelagic geography like Indonesia, other non-medical problems challenge stroke rehabilitation. Especially in rural areas, patients' access to rehabilitation services is limited by transportation issues and long queue times that are due to the imbalance between the number of health workers and rehabilitation facilities and that of patients. To overcome this problem and meet the necessary repetition and intensity of post-stroke exercise, patients must exercise at home. Two home programs are safe and allow for increase in the intensity and repetition of the exercises, thereby improving the neuroplasticity process and supporting optimal recovery of upper limb function. These are the Graded Repetitive Arm Supplementary Program (GRASP) and modified Constraint-Induced Movement Therapy (mCIMT).

The GRASP was formally developed by Harris, Eng, Miller, and Dawson in 2009. It is a self-administered bilateral upper limb exercise that aims to increase the frequency and intensity of upper limb therapeutic activities. Using a range of activities, it improves the functional use and strength of the stroke-affected upper limb by employing low-cost equipment (theraputty, hand gripper, and wrist weights) and everyday items (e.g., wooden blocks, bath towel, pegs, knives, and forks) [9]. Previous studies have shown that the effect size of the GRASP is 0.45, which is similar to the effect size of CIMT (0.53). Furthermore, there were no unexpected events, and the dropout rate was low (9%) during the study [7]. Therefore, the GRASP seems feasible for a wide range of individuals, especially because no wrist or hand movement is required. In contrast, CIMT requires 20° of active wrist movement and 10° of finger movement. This requirement results in the eligibility of only a small number of individuals admitted to rehabilitation units (10%), compared to those eligible for the GRASP (40%) [7].

In unilateral upper limb exercises, such as those prescribed by CIMT and Forced Use, training is restricted to the most affected arm. The basis for unilateral training was derived from Edward Taub's research, which involved deafferented monkeys and was based on the behavioural theory of "learned non-use" of the affected limb [10]. The original CIMT requires six or more hours for therapy and constraint of the intact arm for 90% of the waking hours per day for 2 weeks. Researchers have observed that such a schedule is exhaustive and could lead to poor compliance.

Modified CIMT (mCIMT), a shorter and simpler version of CIMT, was developed to address these issues [11]. This version differs from CIMT in the reduced amount of time and/or intensity of training, as well as reduced time during which the non-paretic upper limb is restrained [12]. For example, a previous study of mCIMT required subjects to wear a "mitt" on the uninvolved hand for 6 to 7 hours of the day for 4 consecutive weeks [13]. Another study used a mitt for 5 hours and provided a 1-hour therapy session at the rehabilitation clinic 5 days per week for 4 weeks [14].

A strong relationship exists between upper limb function and the ability to perform activities of daily living (ADL), as well as social and recreational activities. All are associated with the severity of disability and quality of life; worsened disability leads to reduced quality of life [7, 8]. Therefore, finding the most appropriate rehabilitation program for upper limb function in stroke patients is imperative. Despite the perceived benefits of mCIMT programs for upper limb function, they have their limitation such as poor patient's compliance due to the constraining of the healthy side for long period of time [7]. Therefore, this study aimed to compare the effectiveness of the GRASP with that of mCIMT exercise on upper limb function in subacute phase ischemic stroke patients. It was hypothesized that GRASP exercise could be as effective as mCIMT exercise.

Materials and Methods

This randomized controlled trial consecutively recruited subacute phase subjects who presented with ischemic stroke with hemiparesis. Using a computerized random numbers generator (Random Sample Generator®), the subjects were placed into the GRASP group or mCIMT group. The study was conducted in Cipto Mangunkusumo Teaching Hospital, Jakarta, Indonesia, from July 2018 to July 2019. Subjects were eligible if they had ischemic stroke for the first time, had subacute phase stroke (from 14 days until 6 months after onset) with hemiparesis, and had subsequent mild to moderate impairment of arm function (Fugl-Meyer Assessment Upper Extremity [FMA-UE] score of 26 to 45; could perform 20° wrist extension, 10° active thumb abduction or extension, and 10° extension of two additional fingers). Subjects with receptive aphasia, cognitive disorder (Montreal Cognitive Assessment

Indonesian Version [MoCA-Ina] < 26), uncorrected vision disorder, balancing disorder, and the inability to sit independently more than 2 hours were excluded from this study since these conditions would hamper the subject's ability to comprehend and execute the prescribed programs. Subjects who did not do exercise more than three times would be dropped out of the study. An a-priori sample size calculation was performed using a formula comparing the means of two independent populations and resulted in a minimal sample size of 8 per intervention group. A total of 18 samples were included to account for a 10% drop-out rate [7, 14, 15].

The training lasted 40 to 60 minutes a session, 6 days per week for 4 weeks. Because their FMA-UE scores ranged from 26 to 45, the GRASP group were prescribed level 2 GRASP exercises, which place a greater emphasis on bilateral activities. The mCIMT group used a mitt for 6 waking hours per day on the healthy side and did four repetitive, task-specific activities. Each activity was performed for 10 to 15 minutes. The activities for this group, which included cutting, pouring water, arranging coins, and playing with a pegboard, were unilaterally focused. The participants were required to fill out a log sheet that was included in each exercise book to track their adherence to the prescribed programs. They were reminded daily and told to visit outpatient medical rehabilitation clinics, where their adherence to the prescribed programs was evaluated [7, 13, 16].

The research protocol passed an ethical review by the Research Ethics Commission of the Faculty of Medicine, University of Indonesia (0260/UN2.F1/ETIK/2018). This study was conducted following ethical norms, and informed consent, the benefits, and the procedures of the study were explained to all subjects.

The outcomes were measured using the FMA-UE and Chedoke Arm and Hand Activity Inventory-13 Items (CAHAI-13). The FMA-UE is the 66-point upper-extremity section of the FMA. It consists of 33 items that are scored on a 3-point ordinal scale (0: cannot perform; 1: can perform partially; 2: can perform fully) [17]. Minimal clinically important difference (MCID) values between 4.25 and 7.25 points are representative of clinically important changes [18].

The CAHAI-13 is a tool used to evaluate the function of the hemiparetic upper limb in completing ADL. Tasks involve the use of both upper limbs (e.g., opening a jar, pouring a glass of water, buttoning five buttons, zipping a zipper) since the majority of ADL require bilateral upper limb function. All 13 items are scored using a 7-point quantitative scale. Total scores are obtained by summing the item scores and thus range from 13 to 91, with higher scores indicating better overall function. The MCID value is estimated to be 6.3 CAHAI points [19]. Patients' outcomes were assessed three times by a trained medical doctor: before intervention/baseline assessment (T0), after 2 weeks (T1), and after 4 weeks (T2).

Dominance of hand was assessed by a trained medical doctor using the Edinburgh Handedness Inventory-Short Form (EHI-SF) to measure the laterality quotient (LQ) score. The LQ score was divided into three categories: left-handed (LH) score, -100 to -61; mixed-handed (MH) score, -60 to 60; and right-handed (RH) score, 61 to 100 [20].

The data were collected and analysed using Statistical Package for the Social Sciences (SPSS) version 20.0. The numerical data normality test was performed using the Shapiro–Wilk test. If they were normally distributed, the change scores were examined by paired T-tests within each group and with independent T-tests between groups. Data that were not normally distributed within-group were analysed using the Wilcoxon test, and those that were abnormally distributed between-group were analysed using the Mann-Whitney test. Statistical significance was set at $p \leq 0.05$.

Results

Between July 2018 and July 2019, 58 subjects were screened for inclusion, and 40 were excluded (reasons of exclusion are outlined in Figure 1). A total of 18 subjects fulfilled the inclusion and exclusion criteria. The subjects were divided into two groups: 9 in the GRASP group and 9 in the mCIMT group. No dropouts occurred during the study period, and all the subjects completed the intervention. Furthermore, no data were missing.

Based on the descriptive characteristics (Table 1) at baseline, no significant difference was found between the two groups in age ($p = 0.656$) or the time from the stroke to the study start date ($p = 0.713$). All subjects were right-handed before stroke, and both groups were dominated by right hemiparesis. Other characteristics are shown in Table 1.

Both groups improved during the intervention period (Table 2). Significant differences were found within the groups in terms of the FMA-UE score; the mean difference (MD) between baseline and after 4 weeks of intervention was 8.67 ± 4.47 ($p < 0.001$) in the GRASP group and 8.56 ± 2.07 ($p < 0.001$) in the CIMT group. This result was clinically significant (FMA-UE MCID = 4.25 to 7.25 points). Significant differences were also found within the groups regarding the CAHAI score. The MD between baseline and after 4 weeks was 13.44 ± 4.85 ($p = 0.008$) in the GRASP group and 10.11 ± 2.62 ($p < 0.001$) in the mCIMT group, and this result was also clinically significant (CAHAI MCID = 6.3 points). No significant differences were found between the GRASP group and the mCIMT group after 4 weeks of intervention in terms of the FMA-UE score ($p = 0.489$) or CAHAI score ($p = 0.088$).

Before the stroke, all the patients (100%) in both groups were right-handed, but after the stroke, the handedness category of some of the patients changed. In the GRASP group, two (22.2%) patients became left-handed, and four (44.4%) patients became mixed-handed. In the mCIMT group, five (55.6%) patients became left-handed, and three (33.3%) patients became mixed-handed. Three patients were still right-handed in the GRASP group (33.3%), and one (11.1%) patient was still right-handed in the mCIMT group (Table 3).

Table 1. Baseline characteristics of subjects

Characteristic	**Group**	
	GRASP (n = 9)	**mCIMT (n = 9)**
Age (years)	52.00 ± 4.90	50.67 ± 7.33
Sex		
Male	6 (66.7%)	3 (33.3%)
Female	3 (33.3%)	6 (66.7%)
Occupation		
Staff	3 (33.3%)	3 (33.3%)
Entepreneur	2 (22.2%)	3 (33.3%)
Retired	0 (0.0%)	0 (0.0%)
Unemployment	4 (44.4%)	3 (33.3%)
Education		
Low	1 (11.1%)	0 (0%)
Moderate	5 (55.6%)	6 (66.7%)
High	3 (33.3%)	3 (33.3%)
Hemiparesis		
Right	8 (88.9%)	6 (66.7%)
Left	1 (11.1%)	3 (33.3%)
Time poststroke to study start date (days)	19.11 ± 2.37	19.78 ± 4.79
Handedness before exercise (n%)		
Right-handed	9 (100%)	9 (100%)
Left-handed	0 (0%)	0 (0%)
Mixed-handed	0 (0%)	0 (0%)

Values are mean ± SD unless otherwise stated.

Table 2. Improvements of Fugl-Meyer Upper Extremity (FMA-UE), Chedoke Arm and Hand Activity Inventory (CAHAI)

Parameter	**GRASP group (n = 9)**		**mCIMT group (n = 9)**		**Change**		
	Mean ± SD (95% CI)	***p*-value**	**Mean ± SD (95% CI)**	***p*-value**	**GRASP group Mean ± SD (95% CI)**	**mCIMT group Mean ± SD (95% CI)**	***p*-value**
FMA-UE							
Baseline (T0)	36.22 ± 4.09 (33.09-39.36)		37.44 ± 4.39 (34.07-40.82)				
After 2 weeks (T1)	39.89 ± 4.14 (36.71-43.07)	<0.001[a]	40.56 ± 4.50 (37.09-44.02)	<0.001[a]	3.67 ± 1.94 (2.18-5.16)	3.11 ± 1.54 (1.93-4.29)	0.510[c]
After 4 weeks (T2)	44.89 ± 5.23 (40.87-48.91)	<0.001[a]	46.00 ± 4.69 (42.39-49.61)	<0.001[a]	8.67 ± 4.47 (5.23-12.10)	8.56 ± 2.07 (6.97-10.14)	0.489[d]
CAHAI							
Baseline (T0)	34.78 ± 2.86 (32.58-36.98)		38.89 ± 4.48 (35.44-42.33)				
After 2 weeks (T1)	40.11 ± 4.48 (36.66-43.56)	0.007[b]	42.00 ± 4.18 (38.78-45.22)	<0.001[a]	5.33 ± 3.46 (2.67–7.99)	3.11 ± 1.27 (2.13-4.09)	0.050[d]
After 4 weeks (T2)	48.22 ± 5.33 (44.12-52.32)	0.008[b]	49.00 ± 4.82 (45.29-52.71)	<0.001[a]	13.44 ± 4.85 (9.71-17.17)	10.11 ± 2.62 (8.09-12.12)	0.088[c]

a) = Paired T-test, b) = Wilcoxon test, c) = Independent T-test, d) = Mann-Whitney test. Statistically significant if $p < 0.05$.

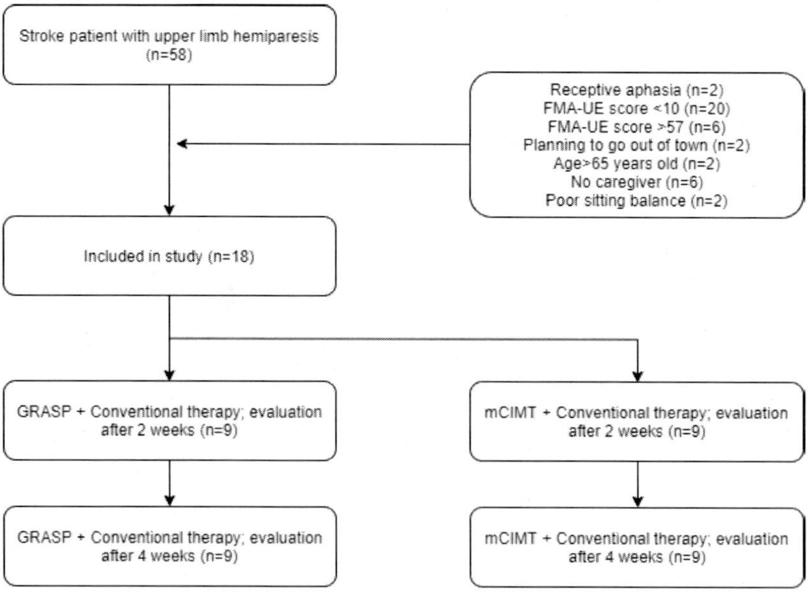

Figure 1. Subject selection flow.

Table 3. Changing of handedness category

Handedness	GRASP group (n = 9)		mCIMT group (n = 9)	
	Before stroke	**After stroke**	**Before stroke**	**After stroke**
Right-handed	9 (100%)	3 (33.3%)	9 (100%)	1 (11.1%)
Left-handed	0 (0%)	2 (22.2%)	0 (0%)	5 (55.6%)
Mixed-handed	0 (0%)	4 (44.4%)	0 (0%)	3 (33.3%)

Discussion

This study compared the effects of GRASP bilateral and mCIMT unilateral exercise on upper-limb motor function and the ability to perform ADL. No significant difference was found between the two groups in terms of upper limb motor function as assessed by the FMA-UE after 2 weeks (p = 0.510) and 4 weeks of intervention (p = 0.489). Furthermore, no significant difference was found between the two groups when the performance of the paretic upper limb when completing ADL was evaluated with CAHAI after 2 weeks (p = 0.50) and 4 weeks of intervention (p = 0.088). Thus, the results showed that both GRASP bilateral exercise and mCIMT are effective for improving upper limb function in ADL.

Improvements were found within-group after 4 weeks of intervention; the FMA-UE MD changed 8.67 ± 4.47 in the GRASP group and 8.56 ± 2.07 in mCIMT group, and both group results exceeded the FMA-UE MCID (4.25 to 7.5 points). The CAHAI MD changed 13.44 ± 4.85 in the GRASP group and 10.11 ± 2.62 in the mCIMT group, and both group results exceeded the CAHAI MCID (6.3 points). These results indicated that the training was associated with clinically meaningful improvements and may help improve upper extremity function in stroke patients [18, 19].

Both groups received the same amount of training time. The difference between groups was wearing a mitt for 6 hours per day during active time 6 days per week in the mCIMT group (the GRASP group was not restrained) and a focus on unilateral and bilateral exercises in the mCIMT and GRASP groups, respectively [21]. The severity of upper limb function before intervention, the time of intervention post-stroke, and the age of the patient also influence the process of neuroplasticity. To meet these conditions, the groups were given the same amount of training time, as mentioned above, and only patients with moderate upper limb impairment (FMA-UE score between

26 and 45); those in the sub-acute phase (between 2 weeks and 6 months post-stroke); and those without significant difference between the baseline time post-stroke to study start date ($p = 0.713$) and without significant difference in age ($p = 0.656$) were included in the study [12, 22].

Although a recent systematic review showed the superior effect of mCIMT over traditional rehabilitation, the variability of the included studies meant that a definitive conclusion could not be drawn [6]. Furthermore, the review did not specifically compare the effectiveness of GRASP bilateral exercises to mCIMT unilateral exercises, but other bilateral exercises with unilateral exercises, such as mCIMT/CIMT. They found that bilateral and unilateral exercises were similarly effective, which agreed with the findings of the current study. Morris et al., (2009) also found that bilateral training was no more effective than unilateral training, and in terms of overall improvement indexterity, their bilateral training group improved less significantly [24]. However, intervention success may largely be influenced by the severity of upper limb paresis and the time of intervention post-stroke [12].

Brunner et al., (2012) also found no significant difference between bilateral training and mCIMT when studying ischemic or subacute haemorrhagic stroke patients after the first stroke or with previous strokes that did not leave any residual disability [21]. In contrast, the current study only included ischemic stroke patients, because the recovery prognosis of the two types of stroke is different. Brunner et al., found that patients with intracerebral haemorrhage had greater functional impairment than cerebral infarction patients at admission but made greater gains [23].

Stoykov et al., (2009) found significant differences between the bilateral and unilateral groups in terms of functional improvement as measured by the Motor Assessment Scale (MAS) Upper Arm Function subscale ($p = 0.021$). The bilateral group had a higher mean change than the unilateral group, but no significant differences were found between the groups for any other MAS subscale, including advanced hand activities, hand movements, and upper limb items (all $p > 0.05$). Both bilateral and unilateral treatments, such as CIMT or mCIMT exercise, were efficacious for moderately impaired chronic stroke survivors in the subacute phase post-stroke [25].

Bilateral training improves motor function after stroke by exploiting uncrossed pathways, including intercallosal connections, and contributing to the normalization of inhibitory influences between the hemispheres. Motor function of the affected arm could also be facilitated by symmetry constraint by a mechanical coupling of both arms applied in synchronous bilateral training [21]. Bilateral arm training is also functionally superior because people naturally use both arms in a coordinated manner while performing various ADL [26]. Because the neuronal mechanisms of bimanual movements differ from those of unimanual movements, bimanual exercise should always be included when retraining motor function post-stroke [21].

In mCIMT, transcallosally mediated effects might also contribute to neuronal mechanisms. As interhemispheric inhibition could be present in stroke patients with intact transcallosal connections, the immobilization of the healthy arm during constraint-induced therapy has been associated with reduced excitability of the healthy primary motor cortex, which may, in turn, lead to a disinhibitory effect on the affected primary motor cortex [27].

Interestingly, before stroke, all the current study's patients were right-handed, but this handedness changed after stroke in both groups. In the GRASP group, two became left-handed, and four patients became mixed-handed. In the mCIMT group, five patients became left-handed, and three patients became mixed-handed. Those whose dominant hand was affected by the stroke may have been more motivated to use their dominant hand during recovery, while those whose non-dominant hand was affected might have little to no motivation to use the affected hand in daily tasks.

Conclusion

In the light of these data, hemiparesis could influence the changes to handedness. This study suggested that GRASP bilateral exercise provides the same benefit and is more comfortable than mCIMT unilateral exercise. Thus, most patients in the subacute phase after stroke do not need to constrain their hand using a mitt. Furthermore, the focus of therapy should not only be on the affected upper limb but should also include bilateral exercise, since ADL are usually performed with both upper limbs.

The limitations of this study were its relatively short intervention and follow-up time and lack of data on the extent of infarction, which could, in part, influence upper limb function prognosis. Several potential biases also existed, including onset of stroke, innate adaptive mechanism of each participant, and the dominant hand impairment. Thus, further studies with longer follow-up and larger sample sizes are needed in the future.

Competing Interests

The authors declare no potential conflicts of interest concerning the research, authorship, and/or publication of this article.

Acknowledgments

This article was presented at the 6th International Conference and Exhibition on Indonesian Medical Education and Research Institute (6th ICE on IMERI), Faculty of Medicine, Universitas Indonesia. We thank the 6th ICE on the IMERI committee, who had supported the peer review and manuscript preparation for publication to Nova Science Publishers, Inc.

References

[1] Misbach J., Ali W. Stroke in indonesia: a first large prospective hospital based study of acute stroke in 28 hospitals in indonesia. *J Clin Neurosci.* 2009; 8(3): 245-9.

[2] Badan Penelitian dan Pengembangan Kesehatan Kementerian Kesehatan RI [Body of Research and Development, Ministry of Health Republic of Indonesia]. Riset kesehatan dasar 2018 [*Basic medical research* 2018]. Jakarta: Kementrian Kesehatan RI; 2018.

[3] Brewer L., Horgan F., Hickey A., Williams D. Stroke rehabilitation: recent advances and future therapies. *QJM.* 2013 Jan; 106(1): 11-25.

[4] Alia C., Spalleti C., Lai S., Panarese A., Lamola G., Bertolucci F., et al., Neuroplastic changes following brain ischemia and their contribution to stroke recovery: novel approaches in neurorehabilitation. *Fron Cell Neurosci.* 2017; 11: 76-86.

[5] Zeiler S. R., Krakauer J. W. The interaction between training and plasticity in the poststroke brain. *Curr Opin Neurol.* 2013 Dec; 26(6): 609-16.

[6] Shi Y. X., Tian J. H., Yang K. H., Zhao Y. Modified constraint-induced movement therapy versus traditional rehabilitation in patients with upper-extremity dysfunction after stroke: a systematic review and meta-analysis. *Arch Phys Med Rehabil.* 2011 Jun; 92(6): 972-82.

[7] Harris J. E., Eng J. J., Miller W. C., Dawson A. S. A self-administered graded repetitive arm supplementary program (GRASP) improves arm function during inpatient stroke rehabilitation: a multi-site randomized controlled trial. *Stroke.* 2009 Jun; 40(6): 2123-8.

[8] Cerniauskaite M., Quintas R., Koutsogeorgou E., Meucci P., Sattin D., Leonardi M., et al., Quality-of-life and disability in patients with stroke. *Am J Phys Med Rehabil.* 2012 Feb; 91(13 Suppl 1): S39-47.

[9] Murdolo Y., Brown T., Fielding L., Elliott S., Castles E. Stroke survivors' experiences of using the graded repetitive arm supplementary program (GRASP) in an australian acute hospital setting: a mixed-methods pilot Study. *Aust Occup Ther J.* 2017 Aug; 64(4): 305-13.

[10] Taub E., Miller N. E., Novack T. A., Cook E. W., Fleming W. C., Nepomuceno CS., et al., Technique to improve chronic motor deficit after stroke. *Arch Phys Med Rehabil.* 1993; 74: 347-54.

[11] Yadav R. K., Sharma R., Borah D., Kothari S. Y. Efficacy of modified constraint induced movement therapy in the treatment of hemiparetic upper limb in stroke patients: a randomized controlled trial. *J Clin Diagn Res.* 2016 Nov; 10(11): YC01-YC05.

[12] van Delden A. E., Peper C. E., Beek P. J., Kwakkel G. Unilateral versus bilateral upper limb exercise therapy after stroke: a systematic review." *J Rehabil Med.* 2012; 44: 106-17.

[13] Azab M., Al-Jarrah M., Nazzal M., Maayah M., Samour M. A., Jamous M. Effectiveness of constraint-induced movement therapy (CIMT) as home-based therapy on barthel index in patients with chronic stroke." *Top Stroke Rehabil.* May-Jun 2009; 16(3): 207-11.

[14] Bang D., Shin W., Choi H. Effects of modified constraint-induced movement therapy with trunk restraint in early stroke patients: a single-blinded, randomized, controlled, pilot trial." *NeuroRehabilitation.* 2018; 42: 29-35.

[15] Barzel A., Ketels G., Stark A., Tetzlaff B., Daubmann A., Wegscheider K., et al., Home-based constraint-induced movement therapy for patients with upper limb dysfunction after stroke (HOMECIMT): a cluster-randomised, controlled trial. *Lancet Neurol.* 2015 Sep;14(9):893-902.

[16] Kwakkel G., Veerbeek J. M., van Wegen E. E., Wolf S. L. Constraint-induced movement therapy after stroke. *Lancet Neurol.* 2015; 14: 224-34.

[17] Fugl-Meyer A. R., Jaasko L., Leyman I., Olsson S., Steglind S. The post-stroke hemiplegic patient: a method for evaluation of physical performance. *Scandinav J Rehabil Med.* 1975; 7: 13-31.

[18] Page S. J., Fulk G. D., Boyne P. Clinically important differences for the upper-extremity fugl-meyer scale in people with minimal to moderate impairment due to chronic stroke. *Phys Ther.* 2012; 92: 791-98.

[19] Barreca S. R., Stratford P. W., Masters L. M., Lambert C. L., Griffiths J. Comparing 2 versions of the chedoke arm and hand activity inventory with the action research arm test. *Phys Ther.* 2006; 86: 245-53.

[20] Veale J. F. Edinburgh handedness inventory - short form: a revised version based on confirmatory factor analysis. *Laterality.* 2014; 19: 164-77.

[21] Brunner I. C., Skouen J. S., Strand L. I. Is modified constraint-induced movement therapy more effective than bimanual training in improving arm motor function in the subacute phase post stroke? a randomized controlled trial. *Clin Rehabil.* 2012; 26: 1078-86.

[22] Kleim J. A., Jones T. A. Principles of experience-dependent neural plasticity: implications for rehabilitation after brain damage." *J Speech Lang Hear Res.* 2018; 51: S225-39.

[23] Kelly P. J., Furie K. L., Shafqat S., Rallis N., Chang Y., Stein J. Functional recovery following rehabilitation after haemorrhagic and ischemic stroke." *Arch Phys Med Rehabil.* 2003; 84: 968-72.

[24] Morris J. H., van Wijck F., Joice S., Ogston S. A., Cole I., MacWalter R. S. A comparison of bilateral and unilateral upper-limb task training in early poststroke rehabilitation: a randomized controlled trial. *Arch Phys Med Rehabil.* 2008; 89: 1237-45.

[25] Stoykov M. E., Lewis G. N., Corcos D. M. Comparison of Bilateral and Unilateral Training for Upper Extremity Hemiparesis in Stroke. *Neurorehabil Neural Repair.* 2009; 23: 945-53.

[26] Waller S. M., Whitall J. Bilateral arm training: why and who benefits. *NeuroRehabilitation.* 2008; 23: 29-41.

[27] Liepert J., Miltner W. H., Bauder H., Sommer M., Dettmers C., Taub E., et al., Motor cortex plasticity during constraint-induced movement therapy in stroke patients. *Neurosci Lett.* 1998; 250: 5-8.

Chapter 5

The Relationship between Number of Flight Hours, Eating Habits, and Physical Activity with Dyslipidemia in Civil Aviation in Indonesia during the COVID-19 Pandemic

Erma Rezki Haryati[1,*], Dewi Friska[2] and Syougie[1]

[1]Aviation Medicine Specialist Program, Faculty of Medicine, University of Indonesia, Jakarta, Indonesia

[2]Department of Community Medicine, Faculty of Medicine, University of Indonesia, Jakarta, Indonesia

Abstract

Background: Dyslipidemia is one of the causes of incapacitation during flying tasks. Lifestyle and work environment affect the risk of dyslipidemia. During the COVID-19 pandemic, changes to work patterns could affect the lifestyles of pilots. This chapter determines the factors associated with dyslipidemia in civil pilots in Indonesia during the COVID-19 pandemic.

Methods: A cross-sectional study was conducted involving 178 pilots who received a medical examination at the Aviation Medical Center, Jakarta. Demographic data, eating habits and physical activity were retrieved using a questionnaire. The numbers of flight hours were obtained from the pilots' company logbooks, and lipid profile levels were obtained from laboratory results. Logistic regression analysis was performed to analyze the dominant risk factors associated with dyslipidemia.

[*] Corresponding Author's Email: ermarezkiharyati12@gmail.com.

In: The 6th Annual International Conference …
Editors: M. Maidarti, H. Winarto, C. O. M. Jasirwan et al.
ISBN: 978-1-68507-925-3

Results: The average number of flying hours during the COVID-19 pandemic was 396.07±197.10 hours. The average eating habit score was 64.34±5.31 and the average physical activity score was 15.03±2.10. The number of flight hours is the dominant risk factor associated with dyslipidemia in Indonesian civil pilots during the COVID-19 pandemic, where an increase in the number of flying hours by 0.99 will increase the risk of dyslipidemia. [P = .025; OR = 0.99; 95% CI 0.99-1.00].

Conclusion: The number of flying hours is associated with dyslipidemia in Indonesian civil pilots during the COVID-19 pandemic.

Keywords: dyslipidemia, flight hours, COVID-19, Indonesian pilots, lifestyle

Introduction

Dyslipidemia is one of the risk factors for cardiovascular disease and stroke, with complications of vertigo and syncope symptoms. This condition can increase the risk of sudden incapacitation in flying tasks [1]. Ricaurte (2018) examined the autopsy report of USA pilots who had fatal accidents between April 2013 and March 2016 and found that 214 pilots (84.6%) had cardiovascular disorders and 162 pilots (76%) suffered from coronary heart disease with dyslipidemia as one of the causes [2]. Factors that can affect dyslipidemia include age, genetics, race, smoking, poor diet, lack of physical activity and work environment [3-7]. Chairina (2018) conducted a study of civil pilots in Indonesia and found that those with inappropriate food intake had a two times greater risk of suffering from dyslipidemia [8]. Chen (2010) found that pilots with a total number of flying hours more than 15,000 had higher cholesterol and HDL levels compared to their peers with fewer than 10,000 flight hours [9].

During the COVID-19 pandemic, the daily activities restriction policy affected people's lifestyles. Most studies of the general population found that sedentary lifestyle and unhealthy food consumption increased while physical activity levels decreased [10-14]. It is important to identify and evaluate the impact of the COVID-19 pandemic on Indonesian civil pilots' working patterns and lifestyles because it can help to prevent dyslipidemia risks that affect their performance. This chapter therefore determines the factors associated with dyslipidemia in civil pilots in Indonesia during the COVID-19 pandemic.

Materials and Methods

A cross-sectional study was conducted on 178 civil pilots who performed medical examinations at the Aviation Medical Center on 12-16 July 2021. A consecutive sampling method was used. The inclusion criteria were fixed wings pilots aged 18-65 years with an Airline Transport Pilot Licence (ATPL) or Commercial Pilot Licence (CPL). The exclusion criterion is foreign pilots.

Participants were asked to complete the questionnaire in full; if any parts were left incomplete, the participants were immediately called back to complete it.

The measurement of healthy behaviour in eating habits and physical activity in this chapter adopted the survey questionnaire Assessment of Eating Habits and Lifestyle during the Coronavirus Pandemic in the Middle East and North Africa region. The questionnaire consists of several question domains that were developed based on the Short Food Frequency Questionnaire (FFQ), the International Physical Activity Questionnaire (IPAQ) Short Form and the Copenhagen Psychosocial Questionnaire.

The first domain asks about personal data, which consists of 15 questions (name, gender, age, date of birth, city of living, marital status, number of children, education level, employment status, type and licence numbers, airlines, position in flight, flight routes, flight hours from November 2018 until February 2020, and flight hours from March 2020 until June 2021). The second domain concerns eating patterns, which consists of 19 questions (healthy food choices before and during the pandemic, changes in the amount of food consumption, diet, factors that motivate improvement in eating patterns, the most frequently consumed foods, frequency of eating per/day, breakfast habits, skipping meals, taking supplements and herbs). The physical activity domain consists of eight questions (frequency of exercise, household activities, duration of work in front of a computer, and duration in front of a screen for entertainment).

To make it easier to analyse, scoring was done on several question items from the domains of eating habits and physical activity based on references from various existing sources. The score for each question item was added up according to its domain to obtain an eating habit score and physical activity score. A higher score indicates that the pattern of life or behaviour is healthy.

Validation was carried out on 30 pilots who conducted a medical examination at the Aviation Medical Center on 18-19 May 2021. The validation results obtained a Cronbach's alpha score for eating habits of 0.615 and for physical activity of 0.664, which indicate good reliability.

Flight hours information was collected from the pilots' company logbook. The lipid profile was collected from the medical report (laboratory blood test) that was performed at the Aviation Medical Centre using Tokyo Boeki Biolis 24i and TRX 7010 as the tools.

Statistical analysis was done using SPSS version 26.0 Multivariate analysis was conducted using logistic regression test with the enter method; statistical significance was indicated by a p-value < .05. This chapter passed the ethical review of the Health Research Ethics Committee of the Faculty of Medicine of Indonesia and received approval for data collection from the Aviation Medical Centre, Jakarta.

Results and Discussion

The 178 pilots who participated in this chapter came from eight airlines: Garuda Indonesia, Citilink, Lion Air, Batik Air, Wings Air, Nam Air, Sriwijaya Air and Air Asia. Table 1 shows that 64% of the participants were aged 18-34, the average physical activity score was 15.03 ± 2.10 and the average eating habit score was 64.34 ± 5.31. Most of the subjects had dyslipidemia (89.9%). Most of the subjects had ATPL licences (51.1%), with Flight Officer (FO)/second commander of the aircraft as their position (51.1%) and mixed flight routes (70.2%).

Their average flight hours before the COVID-19 pandemic were 918.6 ± 391.5 hours compared to their average flight hours during the COVID-19 pandemic of 396.1 ± 197.1 hours. The ratio of the flight hours during and before the COVID-19 pandemic was 1:2.3.

Table 1. Demographic characteristics

Variable	Percentage (%)	Mean ± SD
Age		
18-34	114 (64%)	
35-49	51 (28.7%)	
50-65	13 (7.3%)	
Gender		
Male	177 (99.4%)	
Female	1 (0.6%)	

Variable	Percentage (%)	Mean ± SD
Education		
Master's	6 (3.3%)	
University Degree	43 (24.3%)	
Diploma	54 (30.3%)	
High School	75 (42.1%)	
Marital Status		
Single	44 (24.7%)	
Divorced	2 (1.1%)	
Married	132 (74.2%)	
Licence		
CPL	87 (48.9%)	
APTL	91 (51.1%)	
Positions		
FO	91 (51.1%)	
PIC	87 (48.9%)	
Flight Routes		
Domestic	50 (28.1%)	
International	3 (1.7%)	
Mixed	125 (70.2%)	
Physical Activity Score		15.03 ± 2.10
Eating Habit Score		64.34 ± 5.31
Number of Flight Hours Before COVID-19 Pandemic		918.59 ± 391.50
Number of Flight Hours During COVID-19 Pandemic		396.07 ± 197.10
Dyslipidemia		
Yes	160 (89.9%)	
No	18 (10.1%)	

Table 2. The relation between dyslipidemia and number of flight hours, eating habits, physical activity levels

Variable	Dyslipidemia		Confidence Interval 95%	*p*-value
	Yes	No		
Physical Activity Score	14.96±2.12	15.67±1.91	(-0.32-1.74)	.175
Eating Habit Score	64.24±5.22	65.28±6.06	(-1.57-3.65)	.432
Number of Flight Hours During COVID-19 Pandemic	481.77±146.55	386.43±200.06	(-0.59-191.28)	.051

Tables 2 and 3 show relations between dyslipidemia and the demographic data, the number of flight hours during the COVID-19 pandemic, and the pilots' eating habits and physical activity habits.

Table 3. The Relation between dyslipidemia and age, gender, education level, marital status, licence, position and flight routes

Variable	**Dyslipidemia**		**OR**	**Confidence Interval 95%**	***p*-value**
	No	**Yes**			
Age					
18-34	12	102	1	References	
35-49	5	46	0.71	0.08-5.94	.75[Cs]
50-65	1	12	0.76	0.08-7.19	.82[Cs]
Gender					
Male	18	159	1		
Female	0	1	0.00	-	1[f]
Education					
University Degree/ Master's	6	43	1	References	
Diploma	5	49	0.74	0.23-2.34	.60[Cs]
High School	7	68	1.01	0.30-3.37	.98[Cs]
Marital Status					
Single/ Divorced	4	42	1	References	
Married	14	118	0.80	0.25-2.57	.48[f]
License					
CPL	12	75	1	References	
ATPL	6	85	2.27	0.81-6.34	.11[Cs]
Position					
FO	12	79	1	References	
PIC	6	81	2.05	0.73-5.73	.16[Cs]
Flight Routes					
Domestic	4	46	1	References	
International/ Mixed	14	114	0.71	0.22-2.26	.55[Cs]

[Cs]) Chi-square test, [f]) Fisher Test * Recategorisation is done for Education, Marital Status and Flight Routes because there is a cell with 0 (null).

Table 4 shows that the number of flight hours during the COVID-19 pandemic is the dominant factor related to dyslipidemia ($p < .05$). The increasing number of flight hours during the COVID-19 pandemic increases the individual's risk of dyslipidemia (OR = 0.99).

Table 4. The relation between dominant risk factors and dyslipidemia

Variable	B	OR adjusted	Confidence Interval 95%	*p*-value
Activities Score	-0.231	0.79	0.61-1.04	.095
Number of flight hours during COVID-19	-0.003	0.99	0.99-1.00	.025
Licence	1.632	5.11	0.29-91.13	.267
Position	-0.669	0.51	0.023-8.99	.647

In this chapter most of the pilots had dyslipidemia (89.9%). This result is higher than that of Chairina (2018), who found that among 128 Indonesian civil aviators, only 61.7% had dyslipidemia [8]; bigger samples likely affected the result. The average number of flight hours during the COVID-19 pandemic was 396.1 ± 197.1 hours in the period March 2020 to June 2021. This result is identical to Wilson (2020), who found that the flying hours of 79 New Zealand pilots during the COVID-19 pandemic was 7.8±7.3 hours between March 2020 and June 2020 [14]. The differences in the results are determined by the difference in the number of participants and the period observed.

The number of flying hours during the COVID-19 pandemic was the dominant risk factor associated with dyslipidemia. This result is in line with Chen (2010), who explained that the total number of flight hours in China's flight crews has a direct impact on lipid level or indirect impact through body mass increasing [9]. Huang (2013) observed 628 pilots in China and found that the total number of flight hours impacted the blood lipid level [16].

Work environment such as the number of flying hours, flight routes, hypoxia and cosmic radiation increase the risk of dyslipidemia. This condition will induce oxidative stress conditions that can affect lipoprotein changes and lipid metabolism disorders [3, 17, 18]. Oxidative reactions can cause cell membrane damage, increased permeability and apoptotic cell death but the body will compensate by triggering the release of most lipid molecules as an emergency response [16-18].

Our findings show that the physical activity scores were not a risk factor for dyslipidemia in pilots. However, these findings contradict those of Eui (2015), who stated that physical activity influenced the increasing aviator's cholesterol level [p = .055 OR = 0.320] [19]. Likewise, Zhou (2017) found that strenuous physical activity among Wuhai residents in China was associated with dyslipidemia [OR = 0.78, 95% CI 0.62-0.98] [18]. Wilson (2020) found that during the COVID-19 pandemic, the number of pilots' flying hours decreased and there was a decrease in physical activity in the control group [14].

Increased physical activity levels will increase ATP needs that will reduce cholesterol total, LDL and triglyceride and increase HDL [5]. Lipid level response differs depending on the intensity, duration and frequency of physical activity, initial cholesterol level and period of physical activity [20]. Regular physical activity reduces cholesterol and increases cardiovascular endurance [21].

In this study, eating habits were not a risk factor for dyslipidemia. These results contradict the findings of Chairina (2018), who claimed that less nutritional value consumption doubles the risk of dyslipidemia. Additionally, Arjoelinda (2013) found that long flight routes increase the risk of hypercholesterolemia by 32% [4, 8]. Sari (2016) found that Indonesian civil pilots have bad eating habits and low fibre intake due to the lack of knowledge and rarity of fibre in the workplace [22]. The relation between fibre and cholesterol metabolism is linked to the production of bile acid (cholesterol end product) [23]. Mohler (1991) showed that aviators' eating habits are related to the eating time because of their busy schedule [24].

There are some limitations to this chapter. First, the cross-sectional design cannot describe the course of a disease from beginning to end. Second, the assessment of physical activity and eating habits using a questionnaire is subjective, although it is controlled by conducting a validation.

Conclusion

The number of flight hours during the COVID-19 pandemic is the dominant risk factor associated with dyslipidemia in civil aviation in Indonesia during the COVID-19 pandemic.

Competing Interests

No potential conflict of interest was reported by the authors.

Acknowledgment

This article was presented in the 6th International Conference and Exhibition on Indonesian Medical Education and Research Institute (6th ICE on IMERI), Faculty of Medicine, Universitas Indonesia. We thank the 6th ICE on IMERI committee, who had supported the peer-review and manuscript preparation for publication to Nova Science Publishers, Inc.

References

[1] Aman AM, Soewondo P, Soelistijo SA, Arsana PM, Wismandari, Zufri H et al. [Dyslipidemia management guide in Indonesia 2019]. Jakarta: 2019; PB Perkeni.

[2] Ricaurte EM. Reporting incidental medical findings in autopsied US civilian pilots using the AA- IADS system. *CAMI.* 2018; DOT/FAA/AM-18/8.

[3] Mattson MP. Roles of the lipid peroxidation product 4-hydroxynonenal in obesity, the metabolic syndrome, and associated vascular and neurodegenerative disorders. *Exp Gerontol.* 2009; 44(10):625-33.

[4] Arjoelinda R. *Effect of long haul flights to the risk of hypercholesterolemia in civilian pilots in Indonesia* [thesis]. Jakarta: 2013; Universitas Indonesia.

[5] Blongkod FR. *Correlations between lifestyle and dyslipidemia of state junior high school teachers with impaired fasting glucose in Makassar* [thesis]. Makassar: 2017; Hasanudin University.

[6] De Meester F, Watson RR. *Handbook of Lipids in Human Function: Fatty Acids.* 2015: Academic Press and AOCS Press; 1-809.

[7] Zhao R, Xiao D, Fan X, Ge Z, Wang L, Yan T. Epidemiological survey of dyslipidemia in civil pilots in China from 2006 to 2011. *Int J Endocrinol.* 2014; 2014:215076.

[8] Chairina N, Werdhani R, Gathmyr D. Association of total flight hours with lipid blood profiles among civilian pilots in Indonesia. *J Phys Conf Ser.* 2018; 1073(4):1-7.

[9] Chen WR, Yi H, Zhang T, Feng YJ. Study on the association of Apolipoprotein E gene polymorphisms and flight loads with blood lipid levels in civil aircrew members. *Int Conf Bioinform Biomed Eng.* 2010; 30370358:3-6.

[10] Di Renzo L, Gualtieri P, Pivari F, Soldati L, Attinà A, Cinelli G. Eating habits and lifestyle changes during COVID-19 lockdown: An Italian survey. *J Transl Med.* 2020; 18(1):1-15.

[11] Abbas AM, Fathy SK, Fawzy AT, Salem AS, Shawky MS. 2020. The mutual effects of COVID-19 and obesity. *Obes Med.* 2020; 19:100250.

[12] Ardella KB. Health risks due to changes in dietary habit and physical activity level during COVID-19 pandemic. *Jurnal Medika Hutama.* 2020; 2(01):292-7.

[13] Cheikh IL, Osaili TM, Mohamad MN, Al Marzouqi A, Jarrar AH, Zampelas A et al. Assessment of eating habits and lifestyle during Coronavirus 2019 Pandemic in the

Middle East and North Africa Region: A cross-sectional study. *Br J Nutr.* 2021; 126(5): 757-66.

[14] Wilson D, Driller M, Johnston B, Gill N. The effectiveness of a 17-week lifestyle intervention on health behaviors among airline pilots during COVID-19. *J Sport Health Sci.* 2021; 10(3):333-40.

[15] Supriyono M. Risk factors affecting the incidence of coronary heart disease in group of age <45 years old at dr. Kariadi Hospital and Telogorejo Hospital, Semarang. *Indonesia OneSearch*. 2008; 1(2):275-83.

[16] Huang H, Liu J, Feng Y, Chen W. The distribution of Apolipoprotein E gene polymorphism in Chinese civil aircrews, and a possible risk factor to their overweight and dyslipidaemia is cumulative flight time. *Clin Chim Acta.* 2013; 416:36-40.

[17] Grajewski B, Waters MA, Yong LC, Tseng CY, Zivkovich Z, Cassinelli RT. Airline pilot cosmic radiation and circadian disruption exposure assessment from logbooks and company records. *Ann Occup Hyg.* 2011; 55(5):465-75.

[18] Zhou J, Zhou Q, Wang DP. Associations of sedentary behaviour and physical activity with dyslipidaemia. *J Peking Univ Health Sci.* 2017; 49(3):418-23.

[19] Eui YC, Young WL, Hwa SK. The effect of job stress and lifestyle on blood lipid levels in male aircrew personnel. *J Korean Acad Nurs.* 2005; 35(4):672-9.

[20] Adha A. Relationship between physical activity, fat intake and fiber intake with LDL/HDL ratio in client who checking at The Health Laboratory West Sumatra on 2014. *Indonesia OneSearch.* 2014; 1-22.

[21] Vazquez JMM, Alcon JLG, Alvarez JEC. Influence of diet and physical exercise on plasma lipid concentrations in an homogeneous sample of young Spanish air force pilots. *Eur J Appl Physiol.* 1994; 69(1):75-80.

[22] Sari AD, Basuki B, Mariska I, Budiningsih S. Correlation of physical activity and other factors to fruit and vegetable intake among civilian pilots in Indonesia. *Health Sci J Indones.* 2016; 7(2):118-22.

[23] Allyssa F, Khairun N. Effects of dietary fiber to cholesterol level on overweight patients. *Majority.* 2015; 4(8):121-6.

[24] Mohler MH, Mohler SR. Eating habits during layover affect flight performance. *FSF, Human Factor and Aviation Medicine.* 1991; 38(6).

Chapter 6

Patient Characteristics and Satisfaction at a Free Clinic in Rural Indonesia

Najmah Muhammad Kuddah[1,*]
and Syeda Tazkia Noor[2]
[1]Rumah Sehat Dhuafa Free Clinic, Pamekasan, East Java, Indonesia
[2]University of Indonesia, Jakarta, Indonesia

Abstract

Background: The free clinic is a health facility that provides free health care for the community. Most of its system relies on volunteerism and was built by social organisations. Until now, there has been no official report on free clinics in Indonesia. However, one free clinic is located on Madura Island, Indonesia, namely Rumah Sehat Dhuafa (RUHAFA), which is run by a local non-governmental organisation. This study shows baseline data on patient characteristics, their accessibility to healthcare services in general, their satisfaction and their reasons for seeking medical care in the free clinic.

Methods: This cross-sectional study distributed a validated questionnaire to 30 patients who fulfilled the inclusion criteria, were equal to or older than 18 years old and had visited the clinic more than once.

Results: Of all 30 respondents, the majority portrayed a low socioeconomic background with no formal education (16.7%), low income (90.3%) and unemployment (30%). Although most patients had access to health care services, with 66.6% registered with Indonesia's national health insurance, they still went to get treatment at the free clinic. They claimed that their previous health facilities were further away and

* Corresponding Author's Email: najmah.kuddah@gmail.com.

In: The 6th Annual International Conference …
Editors: M. Maidarti, H. Winarto, C. O. M. Jasirwan et al.
ISBN: 978-1-68507-925-3

more challenging to access, 53% and 66.7%, respectively. All patients in the free clinic were either satisfied or very satisfied with its service. Most patients chose the free clinic as their health facility because it was free (93.3%) and provided good service (86.7%).

Conclusion: Free clinics serve a vulnerable population. Therefore, it is essential to ease the burden of health disparities in Indonesia, particularly for the poor in rural areas.

Keywords: free clinic, Indonesia, rural, patient characteristics, patient satisfaction

Introduction

The free clinic is a private non-profit health facility that provides no-cost medical care services, usually for poor or uninsured people managed by a community- or faith-based organisation [1, 2]. Most free clinics are set in the form of primary care, but some are also set as secondary [1], maternal [3], for children [4], or dental care [1]. The service is offered together with pharmaceutical, laboratory and/or mental health services [1]. The existence of free clinics has been reported since the 1960s in the US [5, 6], and a significant rise was observed in the 1970s [7]. Currently, more than 1,000 free clinics are registered in the US, mainly targeting specific communities or areas using volunteer mechanisms [6, 7]. In Indonesia, the movement began in the late 1990s along with the rise of Islamic charity organisations as a community response to social issues after the economic crisis, including the shortage and inequality of healthcare services [8]. There have been no official data on several free clinics in Indonesia. However, based on records from three major Islamic non-governmental organisations (NGOs), which built the most of free clinics, there have been more than 350 free clinics nationally [8].

Rumah Sehat Dhuafa (RUHAFA) is a free clinic that provides primary care services located in Pamekasan, Madura Island, Indonesia. It was built by a local Islamic NGO, named the Cahaya Ummat Pamekasan Foundation, in 2015. Like other Islamic NGOs, the foundation collects public alms from *zakat* (obligated charity for Muslims), *infaq* and *sadaqah* (volunteer donation) and allocates them to fund several social programmes. As RUHAFA is their primary programme, most of their funding is spent on RUHAFA services. The free clinic has been well-received by the community. However, the number of patients keeps growing, as does the need to improve RUHAFA quality of care.

Studies on the patient characteristics of free clinics have been conducted in several countries. In the US, most patients in free clinics are between the age of 18-64, female, uninsured, and low-income [2, 7, 9]. Three quarters of the free clinics target the uninsured population and are located in urban areas [9]. Free clinics are essential in providing a healthcare safety net in the US, as 1 in 4 patients would not seek medical care without the free clinic [7]. A study in New Zealand also showed a similar result, as most patients in the free clinic were 15-45 years old, female and from a low socioeconomic background [10]. However, those studies were conducted in developed countries, whereas Indonesia is a developing country with different problems in its healthcare systems. This study therefore reports the free clinic patient characteristics that are specific to rural areas in Indonesia because studies on patient characteristics are important as the baseline data from which to make improvements [11]. Such data can be used to assess patients' needs [12], type of medical care [13], possible barriers to service delivery [14], patient satisfaction [15], continuity of care [16], etc. Currently, there are no descriptive data on RUHAFA patient characteristics. Therefore, this study aims to understand the patients' characteristics, their accessibility to medical care and to the free clinic, and their satisfaction with service in the free clinic.

Materials and Methods

This study was conducted at the RUHAFA free clinic in Pamekasan, Madura Island. Pamekasan is a small town located in East Java Province, Indonesia. About 14.06% of its population lives below the poverty line. There are 21 public health centres, 16 private primary care clinics and 6 hospitals in Pamekasan [17]. RUHAFA is the first free clinic on the island since it was built in 2015. RUHAFA provides free health services, which include medication, laboratory and radiology examination, general practitioner and sometimes specialist consultation. RUHAFA opens six afternoons a week from Monday to Saturday (18 hours a week) and is staffed with one clinic coordinator, two nurses, one administrator and two volunteer physicians.

This study was a descriptive cross-sectional study, using a self-administered questionnaire in Bahasa. The study was conducted from April to June 2021. A pilot study was conducted first to evaluate the validity and reliability of the questionnaire. The validated questionnaire was used as the final form. Participants who were 18 years old or older and had visited the free clinic more than once were recruited by a research assistant in the waiting room using the convenience sampling method. The research assistant assisted patients to fill in the questionnaire by reading the question and options if the respondent had a special condition, such as illiteracy or visual impairment. Participants were excluded if they were unwilling to participate in this study or were unable to understand Bahasa. All the participants received a consent letter and explanation from the research assistant. Participants who were willing to participate in the study were required to sign the informed consent form. Recruitment of participants with a validated questionnaire was conducted over a one-month period.

A valid questionnaire consisting of 26 items was used to collect information about demographic characteristics, accessibility to medical care, accessibility to the free clinic and patient satisfaction with the service in the free clinic. Demographic questions included gender, age, marital status, education level, employment status, income and expense. Accessibility to medical care in general was assessed based on health insurance ownership, history of disease and past medical facility prior to the free clinic. Accessibility to the free clinic was evaluated based on ways to travel to the free clinic (e.g., on foot, by private vehicle, by public transportation), need for a travel companion, additional travel-related cost, source of information about the free clinic, as well as a comparison of accessibility to the free clinic and other health facilities. The level of satisfaction was evaluated using a Likert scale ranging from 1 (very dissatisfied) to 5 (very satisfied). Reasons for going to the free clinic were listed as nine items, of which participants were required to choose three.

The collected data were analysed using IBM SPSS version 22. A pilot study was conducted to evaluate the validity and reliability of the questionnaire ($p > .05$). Demographic characteristics, accessibility for medical care, accessibility to free clinic and participant satisfaction are presented as frequencies and percentages.

Results and Discussion

A total of 300 patients participated in this study. Over 60% of the participants were female (66.7%), 45-65 years old (63.3%) and married (80%). Most of the participants were high school graduates (43.3%). However, many were unemployed (30%). The majority of participants (90.3%) had a monthly income less than regional minimum wages and had higher expenses than their income. Table 1 shows the sociodemographic characteristics of the participants.

Table 1. Sociodemographic characteristics of the participants (n = 30)

Variables	**Frequency (%)**
Gender	
Male	10 (33.3)
Female	20 (66.7)
Age group (years old)	
18-44	5 (16.7)
45-65	19 (63.3)
> 65	6 (20)
Marital status	
Single	1 (3.3)
Married	24 (80)
Widower	5 (16.7)
Education level	
No formal education	5 (16.7)
Elementary school	9 (30)
Junior high school	2 (6.7)
Senior high school	13 (43.3)
Diploma/University graduate	1 (3.3)
Employment status	
Unemployed	9 (30)
Housewife	8 (26.7)
Pensionary	1 (3.3)
Labourer	5 (16.7)
Others	3 (10)
Income	
<Rp 500,000	19 (63.6)
Rp 500,000 - Rp 1,000,000	8 (26.7)
Rp 1,000,000 - Rp 2,000,000	3 (10)
Expense	
<Rp 500,000	11 (36.7)
Rp 500,000 - Rp 1,000,000	11 (36.7)
Rp 1,000,000 - Rp 2,000,000	5 (16.7)
Rp 2,000,000 - Rp 3,000,000	2 (6.7)
Rp 3,000,000 - Rp 4,000,000	1 (3.3)

Table 2 presents the participants' accessibility to health care facilities in general. More than half of the participants (66.6%) were members of Indonesia's National Health Insurance (JKN) and almost half (43.3%) were fully assisted by the government. Of the participants, 53.3% had access to health services (other than free clinic) in their neighbourhood. Although 76.6% of the participants had chronic disease, only 16.7% of took medication regularly. Before coming to the free clinic, 30% of the participants took medication in primary health care. General practitioner and other health worker (20% each, respectively) presented as the second most chosen health facility to visit when they were sick, whereas 20% of participants claimed never been to medical facility before.

Table 2. Accessibility to health care facilities

Variables	Frequency (%)
Health insurance	
National health insurance (JKN)	
Subsidised by the government	13 (43.3)
Self-payment	7 (23.3)
No health insurance	10 (33.3)
Access to other health services	
Yes	16 (53.3)
No	14 (46.7)
History of diseases	
Chronic	23 (76.6)
Non-chronic	7 (23.3)
Regular Medication	
Yes	5 (16.7)
No	25 (83.3)
Previous health services	
Primary health care	9 (30)
General practitioner	6 (20)
Other health worker (midwife/nurse)	6 (20)
Hospital	2 (6.7)
Specialist	1 (3.3)
None	6 (20)

Table 3 shows the participants' accessibility to the free clinics. Most participants walk or drive (83.3%) to the free clinic. Additionally, over 70% of the participants did not need a companion or additional funds to go to the free clinic. Of the participants, 76.7% had known about free clinic for more than a year and 83.3% of them knew about it from a person close to them (family/friends/relatives/neighbour). More than half of the participants claimed that other health care facilities were further (53.3%) and more difficult to access (66.7%) compared to the free clinic. Overall, none of the participants were dissatisfied with the free clinic (see Table 4). The participants mostly chose to seek treatment from the free clinic because it was free of charge (93.3%), provided a good service (86.7%) and had complete facilities (66.7%).

Table 3. Accessibility to the free clinic

Variables	**Frequency (%)**
Transportation	
Walking/private vehicle	25 (83.3)
Public transportation	5 (16.7)
Require a companion	
Yes	8 (26.7)
No	22 (73.3)
Require additional cost	
Yes	8 (26.7)
No	22 (73.3)
Time knowing free clinic	
Less than a year	7 (23.3)
More than a year	23 (76.7)
Source of information	
Family/friends/relatives/neighbour	25 (83.3)
Others	5 (16.7)
Distance to other health care facilities	
Closer than to free clinic	7 (23.3)
Further than to free clinic	16 (53.3)
No difference	7 (23.3)
Easiness to access health care facilities	
Easier than free clinic	2 (6.7)
More difficult than free clinic	20 (66.7)
No difference	8 (6.7)

Table 4. Patient satisfaction and reasons to get treatment at the free clinic

Variables	**Frequency (%)**
Satisfaction rate	
Very dissatisfied	0 (0)
Dissatisfied	0 (0)
Neutral	0 (0)
Satisfied	9 (30)
Very satisfied	21 (70)
Reasons get treatment in free clinic	
Distance	12 (40)
Convenience	19 (63.3)
Good building facilities	10 (33.3)
Complete health facilities	20 (66.7)
Free of charge	28 (93.3)
Good services	26 (86.7)
Inconvenience of previous health services	10 (33.3)
Recommendations from other people	2 (6.7)
Others	1 (3.3)

In this study, the majority of patients in the free clinic were female, 44-65 years old and married, with lower education and income levels. These sociodemographic characteristics represent a vulnerable population who typically benefit from free clinic services, especially in rural areas [1, 2]. This study also reports high patient satisfaction with the free clinic.

Free clinics provide health services for underprivileged populations who are typically uninsured and poor [1]. Previous studies on free clinics are highly developed, especially in the US. While free clinics in the US typically provide health services for the uninsured [1, 2, 7], the free clinic in this study does not limit its services based on insurance ownership. This condition is consistent with the goals of the free clinic to decrease health disparities and reduce the financial burden of the health care system on the population [18].

The characteristics of patients of free clinics in previous studies were varied. Most participants in previous studies were female and aged 19-64 years old [1, 2, 9]. The 2013 Indonesian Basic Health Survey (RISKESDAS) showed that most of the patients in primary health care were female (51.5%), married (71.5%) and had a lower level of education (96.4%) [19]. In accordance with this result, patient characteristics in RUHAFA were also dominated by people who were married and had a low education level. In addition, the majority of patients had low incomes, but their expenses were higher.

Compared with previous studies in other countries, the distinct characteristic of free clinic patients in Indonesia is JKN, which is Indonesian's national health insurance scheme that was launched in 2014. The high percentage of free clinic patients who had insurance complies with the Indonesian government's target to insure all Indonesian citizens by 2019, especially the poor and near-poor population [20]. The majority of participants (53.3%) in free clinics actually had access to health care facilities around their living places. Prior to the free clinic, the community health centre was their first choice of healthcare facility, followed by general practitioners and other health professionals' practice.

Community health centres are primary health services that are covered by JKN and are available in almost every sub-district. However, the participants still preferred the free clinic as their primary care centre because the other health facilities were further away and more difficult to access than the free clinic.

According to the Indonesian National Team for the Acceleration of Poverty Reduction (2018), JKN insurance was still not optimal, especially for poor and near-poor populations in outpatient settings because it can be used only in one registered primary health care centre. In rural areas, that is usually the nearest community health centre. However, the facilities, services and waiting time in community health centres still need improving [20]. Being located in the rural area alone had already created healthcare disparities in Indonesia [21]. Utilisation of primary care centres is much lower in rural than urban areas mainly because of lower education and socioeconomic factors (employment and income) [19, 22].

Transportation, distance and cost are estimated as barriers to accessing medical facilities [14, 19]. Nonfinancial barriers among free clinic patients were associated with poorer general health and levels of stress [23]. However, this study showed different results. Most patients could access the free clinic independently and did not require companions or additional funds. Of the patients in this study, 83.3% could access the free clinic on foot or by driving a private vehicle. The free clinic is located in the centre of the town and easier to access. Therefore, most patients in the free clinic did not experience transportation-related problems, and the free clinic was easier to access than other health facilities.

Another possible barrier raised in a previous study was the chronic condition of the patient [14]. About 73.3% of patients in the free clinic had a chronic disease. However, type of the chronic diseases need to be explored before relating it as a barrier. Because of unstructured records and the limited knowledge of the patients of their diagnosis, chronic diseases as a barrier could not be evaluated more. Nevertheless, patients' health literacy of their disease is essential because it is related to higher physical health function among free clinic patients [12]. Thus, patients' recorded diagnosis and their understanding of it need to be addressed by improving the quality of patient records and health literacy education.

More than three quarters (76.7%) of the participants had known about the free clinics for more than a year. The primary source of information was from family/friends/relatives/neighbours. This finding was similar to Truong et al., (2020), who found that most patients came to free clinics by word of mouth. The free clinic had a minimal budget for advertising, yet it could still reach its total capacity every day [24]. Spreading the free clinic information in the community through community leaders or regular patients was considered adequate.

All patients in the free clinic were either satisfied or very satisfied with its service. This finding is supported by findings in other studies about the high overall satisfaction of medical care in free clinics [7, 13, 15, 24] Reasons for patient satisfaction could be analysed more by exploring their reasons for choosing free clinics as their primary care. The main reason chosen in this study was that it was free of charge. This finding was similar to a previous study that found that the main reason to seek medical treatment in free clinics was affordable health care [24]. The second most frequent reason was good service, which was identified by the competency of medical providers and hospitality. Competency was determined by clear communication and patient health outcomes. Good service impacted not only their overall satisfaction but also patient compliance and continuity of care [15, 16, 24].

Additional reason for patients' satisfaction were the free clinic are convenient and offers complete health facilities. Complete health facilities are defined by the availability of needed prescriptions and laboratory and radiology evaluations, which means most patients felt their health needs were met at the free clinic. Previous studies in the US have shown that prescriptions were the second most important service patients seek at free clinics after primary care service [7]. Convenience was judged based on easy administration and reasonable wait times. The free clinic did not require anything other than an identity card (ID) to register, everyone was welcomed and insurance status was not a requirement of the admission process. The registered patient was given a patient card to be brought to the next visit. This simple process ensured that patients had easier access to medical care. The free clinic opens in the afternoon for about three hours six days a week with a maximum of 20 patients. This time allocation was suitable for the community's comfort and resulted in relatively shorter wait times. Wait time was one of the factors that affected general patient satisfaction [24].

As the first study on patient characteristics in free clinics in Indonesia, this study has several limitations. Because the free clinic was located in a rural area and the participants had low education and economic levels, the previous standardised questionnaire was difficult to use, so we had to develop a more straightforward questionnaire that matched the target condition. Patient satisfaction was only assessed using a Likert scale. Future studies could use a qualitative approach to explore reasons for satisfaction. History of disease was only categorised into two groups, chronic and non-chronic, based on patients' understanding of their disease and the need to take regular visits and medication. The diagnosis written in the medical record based on ICD-10 was not yet implemented in the free clinic.

Conclusion

Although not integrated with the national health system and health insurance, free clinics are essential to diminish health disparities in Indonesia, especially in rural areas. Patient characteristics in the free clinic portrayed a vulnerable population with low education and economic levels. Even though patients had access to health care facilities, they still preferred the free clinic because it was still easier to access than other health care facilities. In addition, an overall high level of satisfaction with the free clinic services was observed. The three main reasons patients choose the free clinic are that it is free of charge, has good benefits and offers complete health facilities.

Competing Interests

The authors reported no conflict of interests.

Acknowledgments

We thank the Cahaya Ummat Pamekasan Foundation for building a free clinic for the community. Furthermore, we thank all the patients in the free clinic who had participated in the study.

This article was presented at the 6th International Conference and Exhibition on Indonesian Medical Education and Research Institute (6th ICE on IMERI), Faculty of Medicine, Universitas Indonesia. We thank the 6th ICE on the IMERI committee, who had supported the peer review and manuscript preparation before submitting it to the journal.

References

[1] Notaro S. J., Khan M., Bryan N., Kim C., Osunero T., Senseng M. G., et al., Analysis of the demographic characteristics and medical conditions of the uninsured utilizing a free clinic. *J Community Health.* 2012;37:501-6.

[2] Keis R. M., DeGeus L. G., Cashman S. B., Savageau J. Characteristics of patients at three free clinics. *J Health Care Poor Underserved.* 2004;15(4):603-17.

[3] Gold K. J., Garrison B., Garrison S., Armbruster P. A novel model for a free clinic for prenatal and infant care in detroit. *Maternal Child Health J.* 2020:24(7):817-22.

[4] LaGrandeur J., Moros M., Dobrick J., Rahimian R., Siyahian A., Tomlinson E., et al., Totshots: an innovative pediatric free clinic providing high patient satisfaction to the underserved. *Fam Med.* 2018;50(10):779-81.

[5] Jerome J. Much more than a clinic: Chicago's free health centers 1968-1972. *Med Anthropol.* 2019;38(6):537-50.

[6] Reynolds H. Y. Free medical clinics: helping indigent patients and dealing with emerging health care needs. *Acad Med.* 2009;84:1434-39.

[7] Gertz A. M., Frank S., Blixen C. E. A survey of patients and providers at free clinics across the United States. *J Community Health.* 2011;36:83-93.

[8] Latief H. Health provision for the poor: Islamic aid and the rise of charitable clinics in Indonesia. *South East Asia Research.* 2011;18(3):503-53.

[9] Nadkarni M. M., Philbrick J. T. Free Clinics: A National Survey. *Am J Med Sci.* 2005;330(1):225-31.

[10] Loh L., Dovey S. Who attends dunedin's free clinic? A study of patients facing cost barriers to primary health care access. *J Prim Health Care.* 2015;(1):16-23.

[11] Rendell N., Lokuge K., Rosewell A., Field E. Factors that influence data use to improve health service delivery in low-and middle-income countries. *Glob Health:Sci Parct.* 2020;8(3):566-81.

[12] Kamimura A., Christensen N., Tabler J., Ashby J., Olson L. M. Patients utilizing a free clinic: Physical and mental health, health literacy, and social support. *J Community Health.* 2013;38: 716-23.

[13] Birs A., Liu X., Nash B., Sullivan S., Garris S., Hardy M., Lee M., et al., Medical care in a free Clinic: A comprehensive evaluation of patient Experience, incentives, and barriers to optimal medical care with consideration of a facility fee. *Cureus.* 2016;8(2).

[14] Mallow J. A., Theeke L. A., Barnes E. R., Whetsel T., Mallow B. K. Free care is not enough: Barriers to attending free clinic visits in a sample of uninsured individuals with diabetes. *Open J Nurs.* 2014 Dec;4(13):912-19.

[15] Kamimura A., Ashby J., Myers K., Nourian M. M., Christensen N. Satisfaction with healthcare services among free clinic patients. *J Community Health.* 2014;40(1):62-72.

[16] Kamimura A., Panahi S., Ahmmad Z., Stoddard M., Weaver S., Ashby J. Continuity of care: Perspectives of uninsured free clinic patients. *JPX.* 2019;6(4):305-10.

[17] Badan Pusat Statistik Pamekasan. Pamekasan Regency in Figures 2021 [Internet]. *Pamekasan, Indonesia: Statistics of Pamekasan regency*; 2021. [cited 2021 Sep 1]. Available from: https://pamekasankab.bps.go.id/publication/2021/02/26/bc9d0f4da7a85b29090e282c/kabupaten-pamekasan-dalam-angka-2021.html.

[18] Worth G., Martin T., Christian R., Palokas M. Free clinic oversight and outcomes in the united states: A scoping review protocol. *JBI Evid Synth.* 2020;18(7):1522-27.

[19] Wulandari R. D., Laksono A. D. Urban-rural disparity: The utilization of primary healthcare centers among elderly in east java, Indonesia. *JAKI.* 2019;7(2):147-54.

[20] Health Policy Plus and National Team for the Acceleration of Poverty Reduction, Indonesia. *Healthcare utilization trends under Indonesia's national health insurance scheme: 2011-2016* [Internet]. Washington, DC: Palladium, Health Policy

Plus; 2018 [cited 2021 Sep 1]. Available from: http://www.healthpolicyplus.com/pubs.cfm?get=8223-10429.

[21] Laksono A. D., Wulandari R. D., Soedirham O. Regional disparities of health center utilization in rural Indonesia. *MJPHM.* 2019;19(1):158-66.

[22] Madyaningrum E., Chuang Y. C., Chuang K. Y. Factors associated with the use of outpatient services among the elderly in Indonesia. *BMC Health Serv Res.* 2018;18(1):707.

[23] Kamimura A., Panahi S., Ahmmad Z., Pye M., Ashby J. Transportation and Other Nonfinancial Barriers Among Uninsured Primary Care Patients. *Health Serv Res Manag Epidemiol.* 2018;5:1-6.

[24] Truong R. D., Kostick N., Vu D., Chen L. Y., Cheung E., Dexter N. Survey on the impact of operational policies and procedures on patient satisfaction at a rural free healthcare clinic in Florida. *Cureus.* 2020 Nov;12(11).

Chapter 7

Hand Dominance, Brain Lateralization, and BDNF Serum Level in Post-Stroke Patients: A Preliminary Study

Herry Hong* **and Widjajalaksmi Kusumaningsih**

Department of Physical Medicine and Rehabilitation,
Faculty of Medicine University of Indonesia, Cipto Mangunkusumo Hospital,
Jakarta, Indonesia

Abstract

Hand dominance plays a major role in functional recovery after stroke, while brain-derived neurotrophic factor (BDNF) is essential in stimulating brain neuroplasticity. This study analyses the role of hand dominance, brain lateralisation, BDNF level in serum and its influence on upper limb function in chronic stroke subjects. This is a preliminary study using a cross-sectional design done in eleven stroke subjects, seven right hemiparesis (RHEM) and four left hemiparesis (LHEM), aged between 47 and 64 years old (57.91 ± 5.431), with an onset from 10 to 91 months (37.64 ± 28.905). Hand dominance was examined using the Edinburgh Handedness Inventory (EHI), BDNF serum level and bilateral hand functions using the Chedoke Arm and Hand Activity Inventory (CAHAI). Before stroke, all subjects were right-handed with an EHI score of 100. After stroke, the EHI scores of the RHEM group ranged from 100 to 87.5 (-9.09-100), MH 2 (28.57%) and RH 5 (71.43%). There was no significant difference between the RHEM and LHEM groups in BDNF level ($p = .364$), EHI ($p = .08$) and CAHAI score ($p = .605$). Based on EHI score, BDNF level and CAHAI score were not significantly different in all groups ($p = .474$, $p = .699$) and RHEM group (dominant

* Corresponding Author's Email: herrymd@gmail.com.

In: The 6th Annual International Conference …
Editors: M. Maidarti, H. Winarto, C. O. M. Jasirwan et al.
ISBN: 978-1-68507-925-3

side) (p = .677, p = .685). Stroke in the RHEM group demonstrated decreased levels of impairment compared to the group whose non-dominant hand was affected. Hemiparesis caused by ischemic stroke either in the dominant or non-dominant side caused no significant effect on upper limb function and BDNF serum level.

Keywords: BDNF serum, hand dominance, lateralization, neuroplasticity, stroke

Introduction

The increase in noncommunicable chronic diseases such as stroke has a significant effect on disability, with 65.5% of all years lived with disabilities in low-income and middle-income countries [1]. Based on the 2018 Indonesian Basic Health Research [2], the prevalence of stroke in Indonesia increased from 7% in 2013 to 10.9% in 2018, with the highest prevalence among those aged 75 years and over (50.2%), comprising 11.0% men and 10.9% women. About 80% of stroke patients experience hemiparesis, and 70-85% of stroke patients experience movement disorders in the upper limbs [3].

Upper limbs are vital for individuals to carry out daily activities, ranging from basic self-care needs to doing work and hobbies. Therefore, stroke patients typically experience problems carrying out their daily activities independently. Only one third of patients with severe upper limb paresis can be fully functional again, and nearly 80% of patients with mild upper limb paresis can return to full functional limbs over their upper limbs [4, 5].

Functional rehabilitation goals of chronic stroke patients always utilise the main recovery property of the central nervous system, namely neuroplasticity. Research has demonstrated that brain-derived neurotrophic factor (BDNF), a member of the neurotrophin family, plays an important role in brain plasticity to overcome the damage. Its action is related to the induction of antiapoptotic mechanisms, reducing the size of the lesion, preventing secondary neuronal death, and promoting neuronal proliferation and differentiation. Recent studies have shown that the amount of neuroplasticity differs between individuals and can be caused by varying serum quantities of BDNF [6].

A previous study on 17 stroke patients showed that hemiparesis can influence the changes of laterality quotient (LQ) scores in stroke patients [8]. The LQ score is a measure of handedness that classified handedness into three categories (C): Left Handed (LH), Mixed Handed (MH), and Right Handed

(RH). Using the Edinburgh Handedness Inventory (EHI-SF) to determine the LQ score, the previous study showed that hemiparesis influenced the LQ scores, where over 80% of patients' LQ scores changed after suffering hemiparesis on the dominant side, even though only one patient (5.9%) changed from RH to LH [7, 8]. Research has shown that handedness can impact recovery in multiple ways. Handedness is also an influential factor in performing daily activities; that is, whether the stroke affected the dominant side and/or the changes of handedness in patients recovering from stroke could affect upper limb function in daily activities. As such, the handedness of the patient must also be evaluated before being given hand exercises for the rehabilitation programme [8, 9].

This is a preliminary study to investigate the effect of hemiparesis (dominant side hemiparesis and non-dominant side hemiparesis) caused by stroke on handedness and overall upper limb function. This study also investigates whether differences in the BDNF level exist in different sides of hemiparesis and its influence on upper limb function. Handedness was evaluated by LQ score tests using the EHI questionnaire (10 items), while upper limb function was evaluated using the Chedoke Arm and Hand Activity Inventory (CAHAI). It is hypothesised that the side of hemiparesis will affect handedness and overall upper limb function, and the data obtained could be useful for future studies in the field of upper limb rehabilitation after stroke.

Materials and Methods

This was a preliminary cross-sectional study with descriptive analysis. Subjects were selected from chronic stroke phase patients who came as outpatients to the Department of Physical Medicine and Rehabilitation at Cipto Mangunkusumo National Teaching Hospital of Faculty of Medicine, University of Indonesia, Jakarta, Indonesia. Patients with ischemic stroke, hemiparesis and Montreal Cognitive Assessment-Indonesia (MOCA-INA) scores ≥ 26 were included in this study.

After ethical approval was received from the Faculty of Medicine, University of Indonesia (Protocol Number 18-07-0818) and all participants had agreed to the written informed consent, they were examined to determine their BDNF serum levels and asked to complete the EHI questionnaire (10-item version) and CAHAI assessment. BDNF serum levels were taken once in the morning before the EHI and CAHAI assessments. The EHI questionnaire was used to determine handedness before (by questioning the subjects) and after stroke handedness (by doing 10 activities according to the EHI questionnaire). This study used CAHAI-13 version [6, 7].

BDNF serum level examination using Enzyme Linked Immunosorbent Assay (ELISA) method, in which 5-10 ml venous blood was taken and refrigerated for 30-45 minutes until frozen. Afterwards, the serum and other blood components were separated using a centrifuge. The serum was frozen at -20oC to -70oC. In the ELISA plate, the diluent assay, standard solution, control and sample were incubated for 2 h. Then, 100 μL of conjugate was added and incubated for 1 h. After that, 200 μL of the substrate solution was added to the sample and incubated for more than 30 minutes (avoid light exposure) before adding 50 ml of the reaction stop solution. It was read at a wavelength of 450 nm (the correction wavelength is 540 or 570 nm).

BDNF level of subjects were divided into three categories: low (< 21,527 pg/ml), average 21,527-25,992 pg/ml) and high (> 25,992 pg/ml) [6].

Assessment of the handedness score was calculated by selecting the subject's preference from the 10 items given (writing, drawing, using scissors, brushing teeth, throwing, using knife without fork, spoon, broom, striking match and opening box/lid). Each preference indicates the subject's hand preference to do the 10 activities. Each activity has its own score for each hand, a score of 2 indicates strongly preferred hand, a score of 1 indicates preferred hand, and no preference between right and left hand was also scored as 1. Handedness score was calculated using the following formula: 100*((right - left) / (right + left)). The classification of LQ score was divided into three: LH (score of -100 to -61), MH (score of -60 to 60), and RH (score of 61 to 100) [7].

The CAHAI-13 is a functional measure with 13 items that are assessed using a 7-point quantitative scale and give a total raw sum of 91 (minimum score is 13 that may be easily converted to a percentage). The 13 items are real-life functional tasks that reflect (1) the domains deemed important by survivors of stroke; (2) bilateral activities; (3) non–gender-specific items; (4) the full range of normative movements, pinches, and grasps; and (5) the various stages of motor recovery poststroke. Accompanied by a detailed instruction manual, the CAHAI-13 may be completed in approximately 25 minutes. Because the internal consistency (0.98) of the measure and the single item factor loadings (range, 0.76-0.96) are high, the CAHAI appears to be assessing a single construct – that is, upper-limb function [10].

After data collection, the subjects were divided into the RHEM and LHEM groups. In each group, data from BDNF level, EHI for LQ and CAHAI scores were compared. Other than the division based on the side of hemiparesis, the subjects were also divided into three groups based on LQ score classification to compare BDNF level and CAHAI score. Based on LQ score after stroke, BDNF level and CAHAI score for subjects with hemiparesis on the dominant side were compared. Analyses were performed using Statistical Package for Social Science (SPSS) version 20.0, with a *p*-value < .05 considered statistically significant.

Results and Discussion

Subject Characteristics

A total of 11 subjects (5 males and 6 females) met the participation criteria and were enrolled in the study. The participants were aged between 47 and 64 years, and all of them were right-hand dominant. Seven patients with right side hemiparesis (RHEM) (aged between 56.57 ± 6.24) and four left side hemiparesis (LHEM) (aged between 60.25 ± 2.99). The onset of stroke in the RHEM group was 29.43 ± 18.036 months, while that in the LHEM group was 52.00 ± 41.255 months (Table 1).

Table 1. Subject characteristics

	RHEM Group	**LHEM group**
Variable	(n = 7)	(n = 4)
Age (year)	56.57 ± 6.24*	60.25 ± 2.99*
Sex		
Male	3 (42.6%)	2 (50%)
Female	4 (57.14%)	2 (50%)
Onset of stroke (months)	29.43 ± 18.036*	52.00 ± 41.255*
EHI before stroke (LQ Score)	100 (RH)	100 (RH)

* Data are presented as mean ± standard deviation (SD).

RHEM: right-sided hemiparesis group; LHEM: left-sided hemiparesis; EHI: Edinburgh Handedness Inventory; RH: right-handed.

BDNF Level, EHI and CAHAI in Both Hemiparesis Groups

BDNF levels in the RHEM group were higher than in the LHEM group (22,914 ± 3,305.933 and 20,822 ± 3,843.533, p = .364). The CAHAI score after stroke was lower in the RHEM group than in the LHEM group (89 and

91, $p = .605$). Based on the LQ score after stroke, there was no LH after stroke in either group. In the RHEM group, the LQ score before stroke was higher than the LQ score after stroke (100 and 87.5) and for the two subjects with mixed hands (28.57%). The LQ score after stroke in the RHEM group was lower than that in the LHEM group (87.5 and 100, $p = .08$) (Table 2).

Table 2. BDNF level, EHI and CAHAI comparison in both hemiparesis groups

Parameter	RHEM Group (n = 7)	LHEM Group (n = 4)	*p*-value
BDNF Level (pg/ml)	22914 ± 3305.933*	20822 ± 3843.533*	.364‡
Low (n, %)	2 (28.57%)	2 (50%)	
Average (n, %)	4 (57.14%)	2 (50%)	
High (n, %)	1 (14.29%)	0	
EHI After Stroke (LQ Score)	87.5 (-9.09-100)†	100	.08**
MH (n, %)	2 (28.57%)	0	
RH (n, %)	5 (71.43%)	0	
CAHAI	89 (73-91)†	91 (39-91)†	.605**

* Data are presented as mean ± standard deviation (SD). † Data are presented as median (maximum-minimum). ‡ Unpaired T test. ** Mann-Whitney test.

RHEM: right-sided hemiparesis; LHEM: left-sided hemiparesis; EHI: Edinburgh Handedness Inventory; LQ: Laterality Quotient; BDNF: Brain-Derived Neurotrophic Factor; MH: mixed handed; RH: right-handed; CAHAI: Chedoke Arm and Hand Activity Inventory.

BDNF Level and CAHAI Based on LQ Score Classification

All patients in the MH after stroke group had an average level of BDNF (23854 ± 2684.177). In the RH after stroke group, the BDNF level was 21,776 ± 3,653.285, which consisted of four patients with low BDNF levels (44.44%), four patients with average BDNF levels (44.44%) and one patient with high BDNF levels (11.11%). The CAHAI score in the MH after stroke group was lower than in the RH after stroke group (82 and 91). However, no statistically significant differences were found in BDNF level and CAHAI score between the MH and RH after stroke groups ($p = .474$, $p = .699$) (Table 3).

Table 3. BDNF level and CAHAI comparison based on EHI classification

Parameter	**RHEM Group**		***p*-value**
	MH (n = 2)	**RH (n = 9)**	
Hemiparesis			
Left (n, %)	0	4 (44.44%)	
Right (n, %)	2 (100%)	5 (55.56%)	
BDNF Level (pg/ml)	23854 ± 2684.177*	21776 ± 3653.284*	.474‡
Low (n, %)	0	4 (44.44%)	
Average (n, %)	2 (100%)	4 (44.44%)	
High (n, %)	0	1 (11.11%)	
CAHAI Score	82 (73-91)†	91 (39-91)†	.699**

* Data are presented as mean ± standard deviation (SD). † Data are presented as median (maximum-minimum). ‡ Unpaired T test. ** Mann-Whitney test.

EHI: Edinburgh Handedness Inventory; LQ: Laterality Quotient; MH: mixed handed; RH: right-handed; BDNF: Brain-Derived Neurotrophic Factor; CAHAI: Chedoke Arm and Hand Activity Inventory.

Table 4. BDNF level and CAHAI score comparison in RHE group

Parameter	**RHEM Group**		***p*-value**
	MH (n = 2)	**RH (n = 5)**	
BDNF Level (pg/ml)	23854 ± 2684.177*	22539 ± 3738.342*	.677‡
Low (n, %)	0	2 (40%)	
Average (n, %)	2 (100%)	2 (40%)	
High (n, %)	0	1 (20%)	
CAHAI Score	82 (73-91)†	89.6 ± 1.342*	.685**

* Data are presented as mean ± standard deviation (SD). † Data are presented as median (maximum-minimum). ‡ Unpaired T test. ** Mann-Whitney test.

EHI: Edinburgh Handedness Inventory; RHEM: right hemiparesis; MH: mixed handed; RH: right-handed; BDNF: Brain-Derived Neurotrophic Factor; CAHAI: Chedoke Arm and Hand Activity Inventory.

BDNF Level and CAHAI in Dominant Side Hemiparesis Group

From the LQ score of RHEM patients (dominant side), the MH after stroke group had higher BDNF levels than the RH after stroke group (23,854 ± 2,684.177 and 22,539 ± 3,738.342, $p = .677$). Based on the CAHAI score, no significant differences were found between the MH and RH groups after stroke (Table 4).

It is widely known that the pattern of human handedness is such that approximately 80-90% of the population is RH, with the remainder being LH, at least in the adult population [12, 13]. Left-hemispheric strokes (54%) are more common than right-hemispheric strokes (46%) and often have worse outcomes than their right-hemispheric counterparts. The incidence of large-vessel ischemic strokes is higher in the left middle cerebral artery distribution, contributing to these hemispheric differences [14]. Consistent with the above study, seven patients (63, 63%) had left hemispheric strokes (RHEM) and four patients (36,36%) had right hemispheric strokes (LHEM).

Right Hemisphere Damage (RHD) patients used their ipsilesional, right, preferred limb more than Left Hemisphere Damage (LHD) patients used their ipsilesional, left, nonpreferred limb. RHD (LHEM) patients used their ipsilesional limb alone approximately four times more frequently than their contralesional limb. In addition, LHD (RHEM) patients used both arms together more than RHD patients, even when the degree of hemiparesis was equivalent between the two groups [15], considering that individuals with the dominant hand affected demonstrated less impairment than those with the non-dominant hand affected [13]. The findings of this study are similar to the results of the LQ scores of the RH group after stroke is more than MH after stroke in patients with RH before stroke. A previous study showed that hemiparesis influenced the LQ scores. Additionally, it is important to know the patient's handedness after a stroke before giving hand exercises for a rehabilitation programme [8].

Paresis on the the dominant side makes it difficult for patients to return to activities. However, the findings showed that seven patients who experienced RHEM (dominant side) had CAHAI scores between 73 and 91, and that there was no significant difference in CAHAI score compared to LHEM patients ($p = .605$). Our findings are like those of another study that found no significant difference in functional improvement between the dominant and non-dominant side hemiplegic groups during three months after stroke using Functional Independent Measure (FIM) [16]. This finding indicates that their bilateral upper limb function is quite good whether the hemiparesis on the dominant or non-dominant side. The patients were able to complete the assigned tasks in the CAHAI examination tool, although some patients carried out modified movements to overcome their impairments. For example, patients used their preferred right hand (paretic side) combined with the non-paretic side to do daily activities. The tendency to keep using paretic hands makes the motor relearning process better because of functional task repetitions and reduces the learned non-use effect by using both hands in daily activities, whereas patients suffering from paretic hands on the non-dominant side may learn non-use, which impairs recovery. This explains the non-significant difference in upper limb function between the dominant and non-dominant paretic groups. Using each upper limb also influences improvement in the CAHAI score because it assesses bilateral hand function [9, 13, 15, 17].

A previous study showed that BDNF serum concentrations had no correlation with post-stroke time, age, quality of life and upper extremity motor function by using Stroke Specific Quality of Life (SS-QOL) [18]. The findings are similar to our results, which found no significant difference in BDNF serum levels between the dominant and non-dominant side hemiparesis groups, between the MH and RH after stroke groups, or between MH and RH after stroke in the dominant side group. No significant differences were found between the groups' CAHAI scores.

This preliminary observational analytic study has limitations in controlling many confounding factors that can influence the result, such as onset of the stroke and other comorbidities and factors that can influence BDNF level (such as physical activities). The small sample size of this study also means that definitive conclusions may be difficult to draw. Because there is no similar study in Indonesia, and other studies on the same topic also have a small sample, this study can be a preliminary study for the basis of future research by other researchers or clinicians.

Conclusion

Hemiparesis caused by ischemic stroke either in the dominant or non-dominant side caused no significant effect on upper limb function and BDNF serum level. The EHI score changes in hemiparesis of the dominant side, and it is important to determine patients' handedness before giving the hand exercise as rehabilitation to maximise upper limb function.

Competing Interests

The authors declare no potential conflicts of interest with respect to the research, authorship and/or publication of this article.

Acknowledgments

This article was presented in the 6th International Conference and Exhibition on Indonesian Medical Education and Research Institute (6th ICE on IMERI), Faculty of Medicine, Universitas Indonesia. We thank the 6th ICE on IMERI committee, who had supported the peer-review and manuscript preparation for publication to Nova Science Publishers, Inc.

References

[1] World Health Orgaization. World report on disability 2011. Geneva: *WHO*; 2011.

[2] Badan Penelitian dan Pengembangan Kesehatan Riset Kesehatan Dasar (RISKESDAS). *Laporan Nasional* [National Report] 2018. Jakarta: Ministry of Health Indonesia; 2018. p.1-220.

[3] Nakayama H, Jorgensen H S, Raaschou H O, Olsen T S. Recovery of upper extremity function in stroke patients. *Arch. Phys. Med. Rehabil.* 1994;75:394–8.

[4] Dromerick A W, Lang C E, Birkenmeier R, Hahn M G, Sahrmann S A, Edwards D F. Relationships between upper-limb functional limitation and self-reported disability 3 months after stroke. *J. Rehabil. Res. Dev.* 2006;43(3):401–8.

[5] Harris J E, Eng J J, Miller W C, Dawson A S. A self-administered graded repetitive arm supplementary program (GRASP) improves arm function during inpatient stroke rehabilitation: a multi-site randomized controlled trial. *Stroke*. 2009;40(6): 2123–8.

[6] Triangto K, Kusumaningsih W, Haris S. *Correlation between brain derived neurotrophic factor (BNDF) serum level and functional morbidity in chronic stroke patients*. Jakarta: Universitas Indonesia; 2018.

[7] Oldfield R C. The assessment and analysis of handedness. *Neuropsychologia.* 1971;9(1):97–113.

[8] Widjajalaksmi K, Hong H. The importance of Edinburgh Handedness Inventory short form to determine handedness in 17 Indonesian stroke patients: a case series." *Neurorehabil. Neural Repair*. 2018;32(12):1089–90.

[9] Liew S L, Garrison K A, Ito K L, Heydari P, Sobhani M, Werner J, et al. Laterality of poststroke cortical motor activity during action observation is related to hemispheric dominance. *Neural Plast*. 2018;28:1-12.

[10] Barreca S, Gowland C K, Stratford P, Huijbregts M, Griffiths J, Torresin W, et al. Development of the Chedoke Arm and Hand Activity Inventory: theoretical constructs, item generation, and selection. *Top Stroke Rehabil*. 2004;11(4):31–42.

[11] Barreca S R, Stratford P W, Lambert C L, Masters L M, Streiner D L. Test-retest reliability, validity, and sensitivity of the Chedoke Arm and Hand Activity Inventory: a new measure of upper-limb function for survivors of stroke. *Arch. Phys. Med. Rehabil.* 2005;86(8):1616–22.

[12] Scharoun S M, Bryden P J. Hand preference, performance abilities, and hand selection in children. *Front Psychol*. 2014;5:1–15.

[13] Haris J E, Eng J J. Individuals with the dominant hand affected following stroke demonstrate less impairment than those with the nondominant hand affected. *Neurorehabil. Neural Repair*. 2006;20(3):380–9.

[14] Hedna V S, Bodhit A N, Ansari S, Falchook A D, Stead L, Heilman K M, et al. Hemispheric differences in ischemic stroke: is left-hemisphere stroke more common? *J. Clin. Neurol*. 2013;9(2):97–102.

[15] Rinehart J K, Singleton R D, Adair J C, Sadek J R, Haaland K Y. Arm use after left or right hemiparesis is influenced by hand preference. *Stroke*. 2009;40:545–50.

[16] Sarikaya P M, Incel N A, Yilmaz A, Cimen O B, Sahin G. Effect of hand dominance on functional status and recovery of hand in stroke patients. *Sci. J. Clin. Med*. 2017; 6(3):39–45.

[17] Raghavan P. Upper limb motor impairment post stroke. *Phys. Med. Rehabil. Clin. North Am.* 2015;26(4):599–610.

[18] Santos G L, Alcantara C C, Silva-Couto M A, Garcia-Salazar L F, Russo T L. Decreased brain-derived neurotrophic factor serum concentrations in chronic post-stroke subjects. *J. Stroke Cerebrovasc. Disc*. 2016;25(12):2968–74.

Chapter 8

Using 3D Modelling Techniques to Improve the Teaching Innovation of Difficult 3D Modelling Anatomical Concepts in a Pandemic Situation

Ria Margiana[1,*], **Ahmad Aulia Jusuf**[2], **Kamila Alawiyah**[1] **and Erika Regina Sasmitra**[1]

[1]Department of Anatomy, Faculty of Medicine University of Indonesia, Jakarta, Indonesia

[2]Department of Histology, Faculty of Medicine University of Indonesia, Jakarta, Indonesia

Abstract

Anatomy is a necessary component of medical education because it is required for the accurate diagnosis of organs and human systems. Moreover, this Covid-19 pandemic requires us to be more creative and innovative in the development of anatomy learning. Therefore, we need a tool for students to easily understand the complex structure of the human body via virtual learning. This study creates a 3D anatomy application. The aim of this pilot study is to show the feasibility and benefits of developing innovative teaching methods. We created a basic design of the material, selecting appropriate graphics and obtaining sample application programmes. The outcome of this anatomy learning technology went through several steps of testing. This trial phase was carried out in stages. First, the application was revised based on feedback from the test team, and the final revision was made with a front page explaining the proposer, institution and storyboard. 3D visualisation, open-source software, and anatomy are some of the terms used in this

---

* Corresponding Author's Email: riamargiana@yahoo.com.

In: The 6th Annual International Conference …
Editors: M. Maidarti, H. Winarto, C. O. M. Jasirwan et al.
ISBN: 978-1-68507-925-3

paper. The app offers convenience for students studying anatomy, allowing them to examine the surface to the deeper structures of the human body layer by layer. A table of contents is provided based on the form of structures in each anatomical region. The user can remove and reassemble any of the structures of the body layer as needed. Overall, the study demonstrates the viability of one method for generating 3D models of the anatomy from actual patient data. The educational materials developed herein could supplement the teaching of complex anatomical regions and aid in the demonstration of anatomic variation among patients.

Keywords: anatomy, 3D modelling, teaching, medical technology, education

Introduction

During the Covid-19 pandemic, which has so far lasted from 2019 until 2021, anatomy learning needs to be more creative and innovative. The pandemic period has demanded that such creativity and innovation be advanced at various levels of medical education in medical schools. As it is still not possible to predict how many years it will take for the pandemic period to end, all activities and goals need to be adapted for online accessibility. Anatomy is an important component of medical education that is vital to achieve all targets of medical competence; it is necessary to develop a basis for accurate diagnosis of problems with human organs and systems [1-3]. Due to the pandemic restrictions, it is not possible to use the cadaver-based learning method that was previously used. Therefore, all learning methods have been moved online (online/network) [4, 5]. Meanwhile, students need three-dimensional (3D) visualisation to learn the connection between the structure and topography. To represent the shape and organisation of various anatomical structures, it is necessary to apply 3D modelling techniques to improve the teaching of anatomical concepts that are difficult to do virtually [6, 7].

This 3D anatomy application programme is expected to produce an innovative application to facilitate the study of anatomy among academics and non-academics. This innovation was motivated by difficulties in the field of education, and the final results were used for education. Overall, the proposed product is a reflection from the results of the obligations of the Tri Dharma (obligations of all state and private high education institution) of education for teaching staff.

The proposer previously conducted an initial study using a module questionnaire in collaboration with module administrators at the medical faculty of the medical education study programme. The results of the initial study identified the students' difficulties, and while the methods set by the manager have generally been very helpful in achieving the competencies expected by students, there are still difficulties in understanding the 3D structure, the connection between the structures and the topography [8]. Although there are various other applications, these applications do not generally follow the learning goals and objectives set by the module and the 2021 SKDI, which have been used as a reference for standarizing medical education programmes in Indonesia. In addition, these application programmes are generally high cost, so not all students can afford them. Therefore, we set the next target goal of this programme to produce an innovative patented 3D anatomy application and IPR to facilitate the academic community in understanding human anatomy in an integrated and detailed manner that is easy to use. The aim of this pilot study is to show the feasibility and benefits of developing innovative teaching methods.

Materials and Methods

This study was conducted at the Department of Anatomy, Faculty of Medicine, University of Indonesia.

Technical Description

This application begins with giving the user a choice of whether to study anatomy through one of the methods: per organ system or by region. After selecting the method to use, the user is presented with a table of contents in the form of a list of structures in each anatomical region/system that will be studied. Users can study anatomy from the surface to the deeper structures layer by layer, which means that the user can remove and reassemble any of the structures as needed.

The application of 3D anatomy offered in this proposal allows students to rotate a structure 360°, thus allowing the user to observe a structure from an anterior, posterior, superior, inferior and even oblique view with different angles. This 3D anatomy application also allows users to understand the connection between structures according to their topography.

Application Objective

The lack of offline (direct) access, limited costs and incompatibility of 3D atlas materials for learning human anatomy in medical education in Indonesia create challenges and obligations for module developers and anatomists to help produce a doctor who has good basic knowledge.

The target of this programme is to create a free 3D anatomy application that is easy to use (user-friendly). A user-friendly system will be able to reach all corners and architectures in Indonesia, who currently have no uniform technological capabilities. Making the application free of charge will make it easier for all students to access without worrying about cost issues.

Technology Aspect

The system aims to complement traditional learning methods of the anatomical system of the human body by presenting 3D images to show the connection between organs and their topography in digital form that can be accessed anywhere and anytime. The application was prepared by creating a basic design of the material, selecting the appropriate graphics, collecting data, and compiling samples of 3D anatomy applications. The system was tested, and feedback was obtained from the proposer team. The sales method was then executed, and final revisions were made along with a front page about the proposer, storyline and team.

Results and Discussion

This innovative product developed herein complements traditional learning methods of the human anatomy system by presenting 3D images to show the relationship between organs and their topography in digital form that can be accessed anywhere and anytime. The COVID-19 pandemic situation requires anatomy learning to be more creative and innovative, as traditional methods cannot be used. The product is very much needed by academics and non-academics to improve their understanding of the world of medicine. This application provides a basis for learning the structure and function of organs and diseases that exist in these tissues/organs and will facilitate the diagnosis of diseases. Figure 1 shows the design/photo of the technology example.

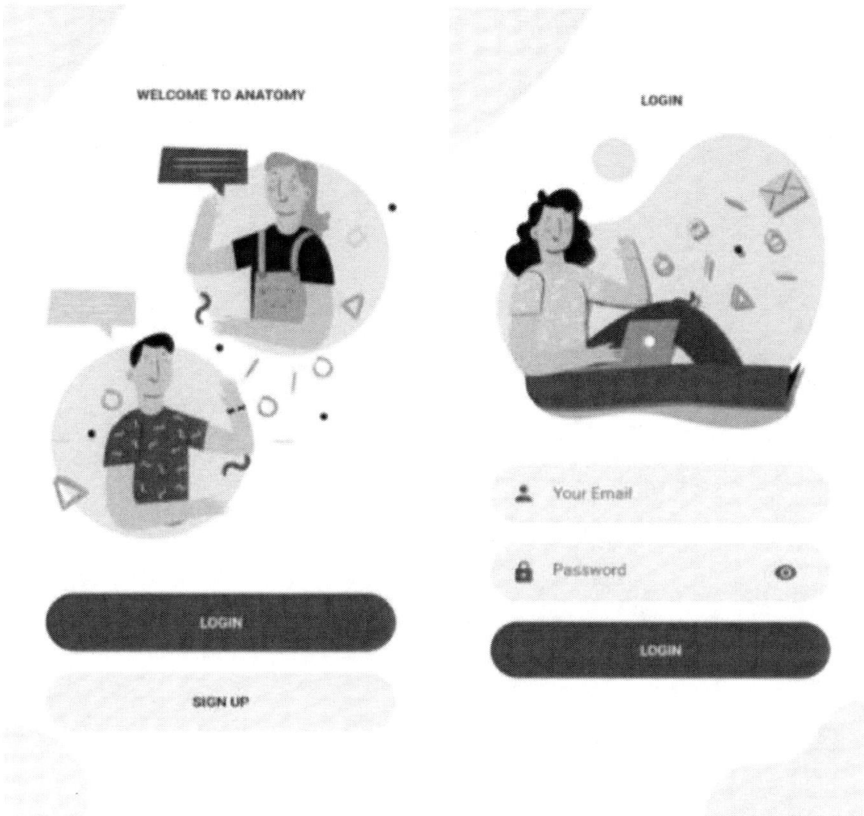

Figure 1. The start and login page to begin the application after installation.

The application consists of categories and courses. The application comprises 5 categories – anatomy, health, medical coding, medical terminology and SPC nursing (Figure 2) – and 26 courses. This technology is available for download and has already been used by several users. This technology presents the anatomy of the body in 3D, which can be opened per layer so that it is easier for users to learn the anatomy of the human body. In addition, this technology provides additional student teaching materials and replaces the use of cadavers used in the traditional offline system.

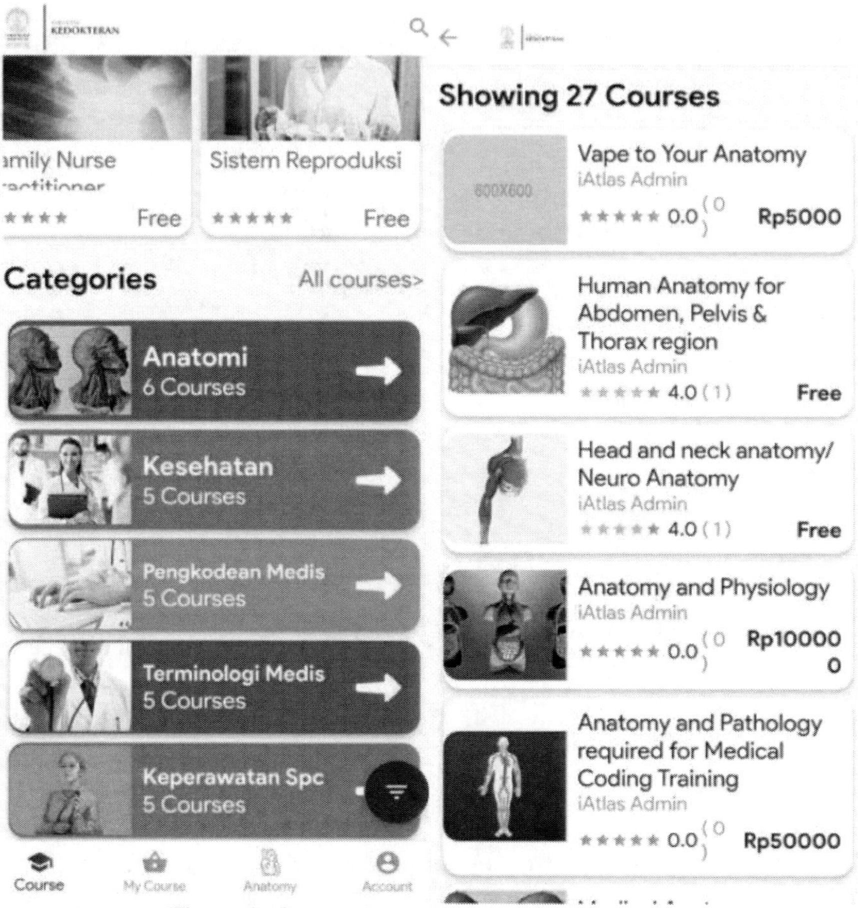

Figure 2. Categories and courses in the application.

After starting the application, the user can select the desired course and category. This application has many functions, which includes learning the structure, function and location of the anatomy of the human body. Figure 3 shows a representative example of an application prototype that can be used. The application can show the location of the structure of the anatomy of the human body and present anatomical structures from the outer surface to the inside of the anatomy of the human body. This application also allows users to open regions of the body's anatomy layer by layer at their own pace.

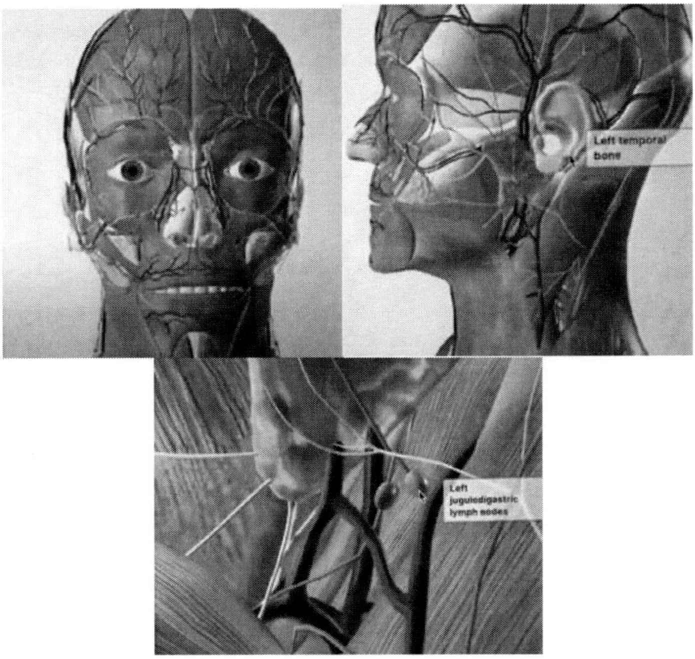

Figure 3. Representation of application prototype results.

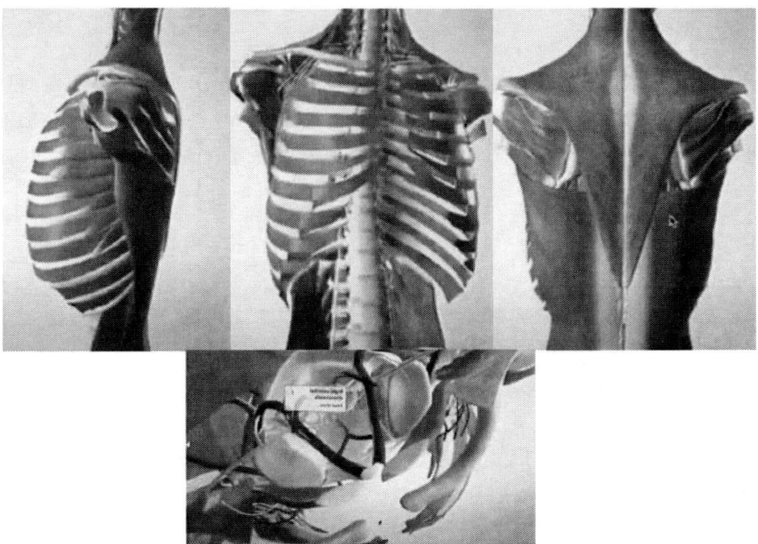

Figure 4. Application prototype of the anatomy of the human body that can be rotated 360 degrees.

Users can rotate the anatomy of the human body by 360 degrees so they can visualize the human body. The display of the application is made with high resolution and will continue to be developed and updated.

Conclusion

This application, consisting of 5 categories and 26 courses, can help students and teaching staff to study the anatomy of the human body efficiently anywhere and anytime in digital form. This application also helps students understand the correlation of each organ and organ system and visualize its position in the human body.

Competing Interests

The author declares no conflicts of interest.

Acknowledgments

This article was presented in the 6th International Conference and Exhibition on Indonesian Medical Education and Research Institute (6th ICE on IMERI), Faculty of Medicine, Universitas Indonesia. We thank the 6th ICE on IMERI committee, who had supported the peer-review and manuscript preparation for publication to Nova Science Publishers, Inc.

References

[1] Chiodini J. Online learning in the time of COVID-19. *Travel Med. Infect. Dis.* 2020;34:101669.
[2] Soni V D. *Global impact of e-learning during COVID 19*. SSRN. 2020.
[3] Fields A J, Hartnett M. Online teaching and learning: COVID-19 special issue. *JOFDL*. 2020;24(1):2.
[4] Vaid S, Kalantar R, Bhandari M. Deep learning COVID-19 detection bias: accuracy through artificial intelligence. *Int. Orthop*. 2020;44:1539–42.
[5] Azer S A, Azer S. 3D anatomy models and impact on learning: a review of the quality of the literature. *Health Prof. Educ*. 2016;2(2):80–98.

[6] Brazina D, Fojtik R, Rombova Z. 3D visualization in teaching anatomy. *Procedia Soc. Behavior Sci.* 2014;143:367–71.

[7] Murgitroyd E, Madurska M, Gonzalez J, Watson A. 3D digital anatomy modelling – practical or pretty?. *Surgeon*. 2015;13(3):177–80.

Chapter 9

Reducing the Risk of Injury in Athletes with Genetic Screening: A Literature Review

Chikih Chikih[1,*], Anggia Prathama[1] and Elina Widiastuti[1]

[1]Sports Medicine Study Programme Faculty of Medicine Universitas Indonesia, Jakarta, Indonesia

Abstract

Introduction: The advancement of genomic research has influenced the development of medical sports science.

This chapter discusses the use of genetic screening to reduce the risk of injury in athletes.

Methods: The literature search was carried out on PubMed and Cochrane from 2015 to 2020 using PRISMA guidelines.

Twenty-two articles met the criteria and showed that genetic markers can be used as prevention for the following types of injuries: stress fracture, Achilles' tendon pathology, anterior cruciate ligament (ACL), muscle injury, plantar fasciitis, patellar tendinopathy, and medial collateral ligament (MCL).

Results and Discussion: The results of this literature review show that genetic screening can be used to reduce the risk of injury in athletes. This finding brings a new paradigm that genetic screening can be used for pre-participation examinations.

Keywords: sports injuries, genetic phenomena, polymorphisms, musculoskeletal injuries

* Corresponding Author's Email: chikih.md.dma@gmail.com.

In: The 6th Annual International Conference …
Editors: M. Maidarti, H. Winarto, C. O. M. Jasirwan et al.
ISBN: 978-1-68507-925-3

Introduction

Advances in DNA sequencing have allowed us to know the genomes of all living things. Utilization of the genome is predicted to increase the effectiveness in the treatment of patients in the medical field [1]. In sports medicine, DNA sequencing can be used to determine the relationship between genetic factors of an athlete with the fitness level, athletic performance, and susceptibility to injury (e.g., musculoskeletal injury) [1]. Genetic and epigenetic influences related to athletic performance are currently highly important factors in much research. To succeed in sports and become an elite athlete, an athlete must have a balance between genetic and epigenetic variation.

The term genetic athlete describes the ability of an athlete to increase their response to physical training (direct effect) and to reduce the risk of injury (indirect effect) [2]. Based on CDC data, approximately 2.7 million sports-related cases presented at the emergency department [3]. These injuries cause losses for an athlete, including time lost ranging from 7 to 21 days, decreased performance, trauma and recurrence [4]. Based on the potential of genomic markers in the field of sports medicine and to reduce the risk of musculoskeletal injury in an athlete, we conducted a systematic review of the literature published in the last five years to determine which gene codes are associated with an increased or reduced risk of musculoskeletal injury in athletes.

Materials and Methods

A literature search was conducted using PRISMA guidelines [5], in peer-reviewed and published digital article databases: Cochrane and PubMed. Identified keywords were either the single use or combination of the following keywords: sport genetic, genetic athlete, genetic marker, athlete, genetic screening, strength, power and sports genomics with Boolean OR and AND. The inclusion and exclusion criteria were (1) article titles and abstracts containing genetic markers and sports injuries that were published between 2015 and 2020, (2) articles that can be accessed in full and in English and (3) articles with all levels of evidence-based medicine with a human subject. The exclusion criteria were (1) seminar articles, (2) articles with a narrative and consensus study design and (3) articles with a case report study design. Category of the research subjects were grouped into 13-44 years. Selected articles were examined by three reviewers, who started by screening the title and the abstract and then reviewing the full manuscript to identify a causal relationship between gene testing performed with musculoskeletal injuries, by looking at the statistical analysis, such as odds ratio, relative risk and p-value ($p < .05$) published in selected manuscripts. If differences of opinion arose between the three reviewers during the title and abstract screening, the article went straight to the complete full-text review with one blinded reviewer, who assisted in the decision-making process. Three reviewers used the Methodological Index for Non-Randomized Studies (MINORS) assessment tool to evaluate the quality of the selected and included studies. Scores of 0, 1 or 2 were assigned to each of the eight assessment categories, with 0 to 6 indicating very low proof of quality, 7 to 10 indicating low quality, 10 to 14 indicating moderate quality, and 15 to 16 indicating good quality. Data extraction was carried out based on the first author, years, study design, genetic biomarkers examined, type of injury, the results of the statistical analysis published in the manuscript and the MINORS score. No statistical analysis or homogeneity tests were carried out in this paper.

Results and Discussion

The two databases, PubMed and Cochrane, were accessed simultaneously on November 24, 2021, using keywords according to method (Table 1). Duplications were removed from the 2,084 articles selected using Covidence. Further selection was carried out based on inclusion and exclusion criteria through the PRISMA mechanism (Figure 1). In the title and abstract screening, 163 articles were excluded because discrepancies were found. These were divided into groups of 65 narrative articles, 33 articles discussing genetic changes after exercise, 5 articles discussing insulin sensitivity, 3 articles discussing return to play, 7 articles discussing the rich plasma palette, 12 articles on examination ethics, 1 examining DNA related to the effects of caffeine, 1 examining DNA related to weight loss and 36 articles discussing the response to aerobic exercise, resistance training and athlete's anthropometry.

After the full-text screening process, 22 articles met the criteria and described the gene examinations performed with musculoskeletal injuries. The 22 articles were assessed for quality using MINORS. The data extracted from the 22 selected articles were author, year, subject, genetic marker, musculoskeletal injury, and MINORS score (Table 2).

Table 1. Search strategy

Database	Key Words	Amount
PubMed	((((((((((sports genetic) OR (athlete genetic)) OR (genetic marker)) AND (athlete)) OR (genetic screening)) AND (athlete)) OR (strength genetic marker)) OR (power genetic marker)) AND (sports)) AND (genomic)) AND (sports genomic)) AND (athlete)	1962
Cochrane	Sports genetic OR athlete genetic OR genetic marker AND athlete OR sports genomic	122

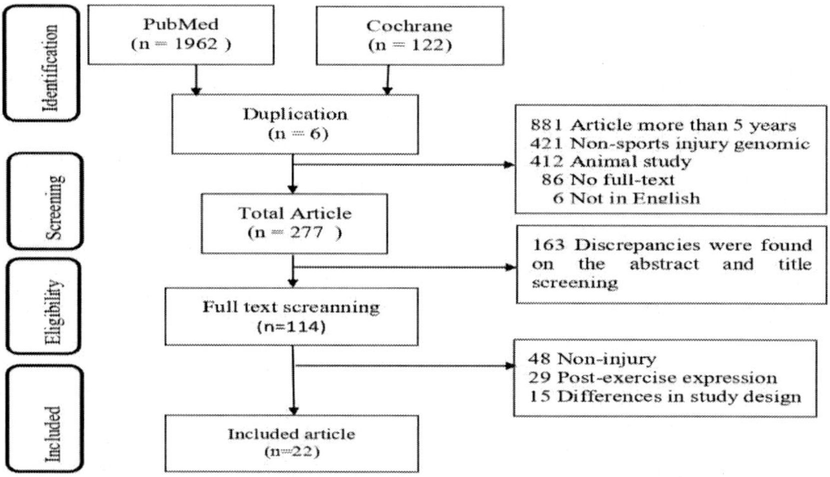

Figure 1. PRISMA Flow Chart.

Anterior Cruciate Ligament (ACL)

Wang et al. [16]. found a relationship between the COL1A1 rs1800012 T allele and the TT genotype as prevention of ACL injury OR = 0.17 (95% CI 0.08-0.35) [16].

Stępień S et al. [14] stated that COLIA1 rs1800012 gene and COL1A1 rs1107946G with homozygous GG were associated with a reduced risk of ACL injury (p = .045) [14].

Table 2. List of study characteristics

Author	Study Design	Subject	Type of Injury	Genetic Marker	MINORS Scores
Varley I[6] 2015	Retrospective cohort	Athlete, Military	Stress fracture	P2X7 receptor gene	11
Stępień S[14] 2016	Case-control	Athlete	ACL rupture	COL1A1 rs1800012 COL1AI rs1107946	11
Karry B[8] 2016	Case-control	Non-athlete	Achilles tendon	COL5A1 CASP8	11
Andrew R[15] 2017	Retrospective cohort	Athlete, Non-athlete	MCL injury	Genome-wide association data	12
Wang C[16] 2017	Meta-analysis	Athlete, Non-athlete	ACL Tendo and ligament injury	COL1A1 rs1800013	15
Shane M[12] 2017	Case-control	Athlete	Soft tissue	COL5A1	14
Pruna R[17] 2017	Cross Sectional	Athlete	Non-contact muscle injury	Gene LIF, CCL2, GEFT, MYF5, DES, HGF, MMP3, GDF5,	11
Juan D C[18] 2017	Case-control	Athlete	Muscle injury	ACTN 3 gene	14
Mustafa K[19] 2017	Systematic-Review	Athlete, Non-Athlete	ACL rupture	Genetic variants base LGC on genomic	15
Varley I[7] 2018	Cohort	Athlete	Stress-Fracture	SOST rs1877632, VDR rs10735810 and rs731236	13
Longo U.G[20] 2018	Case-control	Athlete Non-athlete	Rotator Cuff Tears	COL5A1 rs12722	12
Kim S.K[13] 2018	Cross Sectional	Athlete Non-athlete	Plantar Facial Disorder	Chromosome 5 rs 118704153D and rs62051384	14

Table 2. (Continued)

Author	Study Design	Subject	Type of Injury	Genetic Marker	MINORS Scores
El Khoury[21] 2018	Case-control	Global population	Patella Tendinopathy	TIMP-2 ADAMTS-4	11
Salles J.I[11] 2019	Case-control	Athlete	Tendinopathy	Fc receptor-like 3 gene (FCRL3-169T>C), Forkhead box P3 (FOXP3-2383C>T)	13
Xin-Kang[9] 2019	Case-control	Global population	Achilles Tendinopathy	MPP7, TIMP2, CASP8	11
Massidda M[22] 2019	Case-control	Athlete Non-Athlete	Muscular injury	ACTN3 R577XX, R577RX, R577RR	12
Nie G[10] 2019	Case-control	Global population	Achilles Tendinopathy	MMP3 TIMP2	12
Coelho D B[23] 2019	Cross-sectional	Athlete	Muscle injury	ACTN3 RR/RX or XX	12
Kumagai H[24] 2019	Cross-sectional	Athlete	Muscle injury	ESR1 rs2234693 C/T and rs9340799 G/A	12
Zhao D[25] 2020	Case-control	Global population	ACL injury	COL1A1, COL5A1, COL12A1	12
Seale K[26]	Case-control	Athlete Non-athlete	Rotator cuff tendinopathy, ACL ruptures Carpal tunnel	CASP8	12
Massidda M[27] 2020	Cohort retrospective	Athlete	Muscle Injury	ACE I/D	13

This study contradicts the results of those from Mustafa et al. [19] regarding the relationship between ACL rupture with the COL1A1 rs1800012 and COL3A1 rs1800255 genes because of a lack of evidence [19].

Mustafa et al. found that VEGFA rs1570360 GA genotype increases the risk for ACL rupture [19].

Zhao et al. [25] stated that changes in COLI2A1 rs970547 A allele related to ACL injury OR = 1.8 (p = .019) and with AA genotype increased ACL injury risk OR = 1.61 (p = .026). Additionally, COLI2A1 rs240736, rs1800787, rs1800788, rs1800790 and rs2227389 in the fib-promoter region were associated with ACL injury and it was also influenced by genotype variation [25].

Seale [26] stated that gene CASP8 del-C haplotype rs3834129–rs13113 allele T and rs1045485–rs13113 genotype G-T were significantly associated with ACL rupture (p = .022; p=.028) and non-contact ACL ruptures (p = .036) [26].

Muscular Injury

Jual del Coso et al. [18] found that runners with the ACTN3 gene with genotypes XX and RX had a higher level of muscle damage than those with genotype RR (p = .04) [18]. Massidda M et al. [27] found a significant relationship between the ACE I/D polymorphism and the dominant genotype D for muscle injury among soccer players with OR = 0.48 (95% CI: 0.24–0.97, p = .040) [27].

Massidda [22] also concluded that athletes with ACTN3 577XX gene expression have a higher risk of muscular injury compared to 577RR OR: 2.66(1.09-6.63).

Another finding is that the ACTN3 XX allele had indicating risk of a severe injury OR = 2.13(95% CI: 1.25-3.74, p = .0054) compared with their RR allele, whereas RX allele had 1.63 higher odds of having a severe injury compared with the RR players (95% CI: 1.10-2.40, p = .015) [22]. Coelho et al. [23] concluded that the ACTN3 RR genotype had a higher response to increase creatine kinase and testosterone post-match (p < .05), which is a hormonal stress response to prevent muscle damage compared to the RX genotype [23].

Kumagai et al. [24] stated estrogen receptor gene1 (ESR1) rs22334693 genotype C lowers the risk of muscle injury with OR = 0.70 (95% CI:0.53–0.91) and reduces muscle stiffness more quickly (CC$<$CT$<$TT) allele with $r = 0.135$, $p = .029$ [24]. Other protector genes are HGF rs5745678 T allele, which protects from severe injuries ($p < .002$), and HGF rs5745697 A allele (CA/AA), which protects from moderate injuries ($p < .008$) [17]. Muscle recovery time is faster for HGF genes rs5745678 genotype CT/TT (mean = 19.83 (16.57–23.10) days) compared with genotype CC (mean = 27.72 (23.88–31.57) days) with $p = .009$; HGF rs5745697 allele CA/AA also have faster recovery time (mean = 20.67 (16.96–24.38) days) compared with CC ($p = .02$) [17]. Another genetic marker for recovery time is GEFT rs11613457 genotype GG, which increases recovery time compared to GA genotype ($p < .004$) [17].

Medial Collateral Ligament (MCL)

The GRPEL1 gene on chromosome 4 with the allele variation rs80351309 genotype T related to MCL injuries, OR = 2.12 (95% CI; 1.86-2.38), and the FLJ36777 gene on chromosome 20 genotype C with variations in rs6083471 also related to increased MCL injury risk, OR = 1.57 (95% CI; 142-172), which explains how individual variations affect the risk of MCL injuries [15].

Patellar Tendinopathy

This literature study found that the presence of methylation of the A Disintegrin and Metalloproteinase with Thrombospondin motifs (ADAMTS) gene genotype G at site 3 is associated with the occurrence of patellar tendinopathy ($p = .016$) [21]. While tendinopathy, in general, can increase with age, sex and duration of play risk, it can be amplified by the presence of the FCRL3 –169C gene OR = 1.44 (95% CI = 1.02 – 2.04), FCRL3 – 169TC or – 169CC, and FOXP3 – 2383CT or – 2383TT also increases the risk of tendinopathy among athletes with tendon pain, OR = 2.24(95% CI: 1.14 – 4.40), $p < .05$ [11].

Clinical Implications and Future Research

The findings of this study offer a new paradigm for conducting genetic screening examinations in pre-participation examinations before becoming an elite athlete.

Conclusion

The results of the literature review show that genetic examination in the sports medicine field is still wide open. Several genetic markers can be used for athlete screening, such as (1) P2X7R rs375114, SOST rs1877632 and the VDR gene rs10735810 for a stress fracture, (2) the COL5AI gene and CASPB for Achilles tendon pathology, (3) the COLI2A1 gene for ACL injury and CASP8 del-C for non-contact ACL ruptures, (4) the ACTN3 genotype XX/RX muscle injury and ESR1 genotype T for muscle stiffness, (5) Chromosome 16 rs62051384 genotype T for plantar fasciitis, (6) the ADAMTS gene genotype G for patellar tendinopathy, (7) the GRPEL1 gene on chromosome 4 and the FLJ36777 gene on chromosome 20 for MCL injuries. These findings may bring a new paradigm to injury prevention screening in athletes.

Limitation for Review Process

The review of selected articles among the three authors was not done blinded, indicating higher levels of agreement among the authors.

Limitations of the Included Study

Not all selected articles included clear OR or RR calculations and 95% CI; some articles only had *p*-values, and this search only found two articles that were rated good based on the appraisal we carried out.

Competing Interests

The author declares no conflict of interest and does not accept sponsorship.

Acknowledgment

Thanks to Dr. Nani Cahyani Sudarsono, Sp.KO, as the Head of the Centre for Sports and Exercise Studies, who has provided support, motivation and guidance in the preparation of this paper.

References

[1] Tanisawa K, Wang G, Seto J, Verdouka I, Twycross-Lewis R, Karanikolou A et al. Sport and exercise genomics: the FIMS 2019 consensus statement update. *Br J Sports Med*. 2020 Aug; 54(16):969-75.

[2] Pickering C, Kiely J, Grgic J, Lucia A, Del Coso J. Can genetic testing identify talent for sport? *Genes* (Basel). 2019 Nov 26; 10(12):972.

[3] Rui P, Ashman JJ, Akinseye A. Emergency department visits for injuries sustained during sports and recreational activities by patients aged 5-24 years, 2010-2016. *Natl Health Stat Report.* 2019 Nov; (133):1-15.

[4] Gulbrandsen M, Hartigan DE, Patel KA, Makovicka JL, Tummala SV, Chhabra A. Ten-Year Epidemiology of Ankle Injuries in Men's and Women's Collegiate Soccer Players. *J Athl Train*. 2019 Aug; 54(8):881-8.

[5] Liberati A, Altman DG, Tetzlaff J, Mulrow C, Gøtzsche PC, Ioannidis JP, et al. The PRISMA statement for reporting systematic reviews and meta-analyses of studies that evaluate healthcare interventions: Explanation and elaboration. *BMJ.* 2009 Jul 21; 339:b2700.

[6] Varley I, Greeves JP, Sale C, Friedman E, Moran DS, Yanovich R et al. Functional polymorphisms in the P2X7 receptor gene are associated with stress fracture injury. *Purinergic Signal*. 2016 Mar; 12(1):103-13.

[7] Varley I, Hughes DC, Greeves JP, Stellingwerff T, Ranson C, Fraser WD, Sale C. The association of novel polymorphisms with stress fracture injury in Elite Athletes: Further insights from the SFEA cohort. *J Sci Med Sport.* 2018 Jun; 21(6):564-8.

[8] Brown KL, Seale KB, El Khoury LY, Posthumus M, Ribbans WJ, Raleigh SM, Collins M, September AV. Polymorphisms within the COL5A1 gene and regulators of the extracellular matrix modify the risk of Achilles tendon pathology in a British case-control study. *J Sports Sci.* 2017 Aug; 35(15):1475-83.

[9] Kang X, Tian B, Zhang L, Ge Z, Zhao Y, Zhang Y. Relationship of common variants in MPP7, TIMP2 and CASP8 genes with the risk of chronic achilles tendinopathy. *Sci Rep.* 2019 Nov 26; 9(1):17627.

[10] Nie G, Wen X, Liang X, Zhao H, Li Y, Lu J. Additional evidence supports association of common genetic variants in MMP3 and TIMP2 with increased risk of chronic Achilles tendinopathy susceptibility. *J Sci Med Sport.* 2019 Oct; 22(10):1074-1078.

[11] Salles JI, Lopes LR, Duarte MEL, Morrissey D, Martins MB, Machado DE, Guimarães JAM, Perini JA. Fc receptor-like 3 (-169T>C) polymorphism increases

the risk of tendinopathy in volleyball athletes: A case control study. *BMC Med Genet.* 2018 Jul 18; 19(1):119.

[12] Heffernan SM, Kilduff LP, Erskine RM, Day SH, Stebbings GK, Cook CJ, Raleigh SM, Bennett MA, Wang G, Collins M, Pitsiladis YP, Williams AG. COL5A1 gene variants previously associated with reduced soft tissue injury risk are associated with elite athlete status in rugby. *BMC Genomics.* 2017 Nov 14; 18(Suppl 8):820.

[13] Kim SK, Ioannidis JPA, Ahmed MA, Avins AL, Kleimeyer JP, Fredericson M, Dragoo JL. Two genetic variants associated with plantar fascial disorders. *Int J Sports Med.* 2018 Apr; 39(4):314-21.

[14] Stepien-Slodkowska M, Ficek K, Zietek P, Kaczmarczyk M, Lubkowska W, Szark-Eckardt M, Cieszczyk P. Is the combination of COL1A1 gene polymorphisms a marker of injury risk? *J Sport Rehabil.* 2017 May; 26(3):234-8.

[15] Roos AK, Avins AL, Ahmed MA, Kleimeyer JP, Roos TR, Fredericson M, Ioannidis JPA, Dragoo JL, Kim S. Two genetic loci associated with medial collateral ligament injury. *Int J Sports Med.* 2017 Jul; 38(7):501-7.

[16] Wang C, Li H, Chen K, Wu B, Liu H. Association of polymorphisms rs1800012 in COL1A1 with sports-related tendon and ligament injuries: A meta-analysis. *Oncotarget.* 2017 Apr 18; 8(16):27627-34.

[17] Pruna R, Artells R, Lundblad M, Maffulli N. Genetic biomarkers in non-contact muscle injuries in elite soccer players. *Knee Surg Sports Traumatol Arthrosc.* 2017 Oct; 25(10):3311-3318.

[18] Del Coso J, Valero M, Salinero JJ, Lara B, Díaz G, Gallo-Salazar C, Ruiz-Vicente D, Areces F, Puente C, Carril JC, Cacabelos R. ACTN3 genotype influences exercise-induced muscle damage during a marathon competition. *Eur J Appl Physiol.* 2017 Mar; 117(3):409-16.

[19] Kaynak M, Nijman F, van Meurs J, Reijman M, Meuffels DE. Genetic variants and anterior cruciate ligament rupture: a systematic review. *Sports Med.* 2017 Aug; 47(8):1637-50.

[20] Longo UG, Margiotti K, Petrillo S, Rizzello G, Fusilli C, Maffulli N, De Luca A, Denaro V. Genetics of rotator cuff tears: no association of col5a1 gene in a case-control study. *BMC Med Genet.* 2018 Dec 20; 19(1):217.

[21] El Khoury LY, Rickaby R, Samiric T, Raleigh SM. Promoter methylation status of the TIMP2 and ADAMTS4 genes and patellar tendinopathy. *J Sci Med Sport.* 2018 Apr; 21(4):378-82.

[22] Massidda M, Voisin S, Culigioni C, Piras F, Cugia P, Yan X, Eynon N, Calò CM. ACTN3 R577X Polymorphism is associated with the incidence and severity of injuries in professional football players. *Clin J Sport Med.* 2019 Jan; 29(1):57-61.

[23] Coelho DB, Pimenta EM, Rosse IC, Veneroso C, Pussieldi GA, Becker LK, Oliveira EC, Carvalho MRS, Silami-Garcia E. Alpha-Actinin-3 R577X Polymorphism influences muscle damage and hormonal responses after a soccer game. *J Strength Cond Res.* 2019 Oct; 33(10):2655-64.

[24] Kumagai H, Miyamoto-Mikami E, Hirata K, Kikuchi N, Kamiya N, Hoshikawa S, Zempo H, Naito H, Miyamoto N, Fuku N. ESR1 rs2234693 Polymorphism is associated with muscle injury and muscle stiffness. *Med Sci Sports Exerc.* 2019 Jan; 51(1):19-26.

[25] Zhao D, Zhang Q, Lu Q, Hong C, Luo T, Duan Q, Shu S, Lv J, Zhao W. Correlations between the genetic variations in the COL1A1, COL5A1, COL12A1, and β-fibrinogen genes and anterior cruciate ligament injury in chinese patients[a]. *J Athl Train*. 2020 May; 55(5):515-21.

[26] Seale K, Burger M, Posthumus M, Häger CK, Stattin E, Nilsson KG, Collins M, September AV. The apoptosis pathway and CASP8 variants conferring risk for acute and overuse musculoskeletal injuries. *J Orthop Res*. 2020 Mar; 38(3):680-8.

[27] Massidda M, Miyamoto-Mikami E, Kumagai H, Ikeda H, Shimasaki Y, Yoshimura M, Cugia P, Piras F, Scorcu M, Kikuchi N, Calò CM, Fuku N. Association between the ACE I/D polymorphism and muscle injuries in Italian and Japanese elite football players. *J Sports Sci*. 2020 Nov; 38(21):2423-9.

Chapter 10

Ultrasound-Guided Erector Spinae Plane Block for Surgical Anaesthesia in Percutaneous Nephrolithotomy: A Case Series

Irma Lusiana Tantri[1], Raden Besthadi Sukmono[1,*], Pryambodho[1] and Ponco Birowo[2]

[1]Department of Anesthesiology and Intensive Care, Faculty of Medicine, Universitas Indonesia – Dr Cipto Mangunkusumo National General Hospital, Jakarta, Indonesia
[2]Department of Urology, Faculty of Medicine, Universitas Indonesia – Dr Cipto Mangunkusumo National General Hospital, Jakarta, Indonesia

Abstract

Background: Erector spinae plane (ESP) block is an interfacial block reported to provide adequate postoperative analgesia for abdominal surgery. However, studies on its effectiveness for percutaneous nephrolithotomy (PCNL) are limited. Therefore, this chapter determines the effectiveness of ESP block in providing surgical anaesthesia for patients undergoing PCNL. *Methods:* The study recruited four patients and obtained their informed consent before the procedure. All patients received sedation with propofol and were positioned laterally to receive ultrasound-guided ESP blocks before the procedure. Twenty-five ml of 0.5% bupivacaine with epinephrine 1:200.000 was injected at the T9 level. Before urethral manipulation, patients were given fentanyl 50 mcg intravenously, and sedation was maintained throughout the procedure. The sensory loss was evaluated by performing skin clamping at the incision level before the surgery. The ESP block was considered successful in providing surgical anaesthesia, as there was no movement

* Corresponding Author's Email: besth25@gmail.com.

In: The 6th Annual International Conference …
Editors: M. Maidarti, H. Winarto, C. O. M. Jasirwan et al.
ISBN: 978-1-68507-925-3

or significant changes in vital signs during skin clamping and throughout the surgery. *Results:* The surgical procedures of all four patients were successful. There was no movement or significant change in vital signs during skin clamping or throughout the procedure. *Conclusion:* ESP block is a feasible alternative for providing surgical anaesthesia in patients undergoing PCNL.

Keywords: erector spinae block, surgical anaesthesia, percutaneous nephrolithotomy

Case Series

Introduction

Percutaneous nephrolithotomy (PCNL) is one of the most common surgeries performed to treat renal calculi worldwide. Being a minimally invasive surgery, it excels in having shorter surgery duration and recovery duration [1].

Erector spinae plane (ESP) block is a novel interfacial plane block that has been used widely for pain management on the thoracoabdominal regions since its discovery of having a minimal effect on hemodynamic stability and low incidence of complications. Furthermore, the use of ultrasound may improve its success rate while also reducing the associated risk. However, there is only limited evidence of its applicability in PCNL.

In our institution, the PCNL procedure has been performed under a subarachnoid block. As the most common regional anaesthesia technique in PNCL, this block has some intraoperative complications, such as hypotension, nausea, urinary retention and spinal hematoma [2]. This chapter presents cases of patients undergoing ESP blocks as the surgical anaesthesia technique for PCNL.

Methods

After obtaining approval from the Research Ethics Committee of the Faculty of Medicine, Universitas Indonesia – Cipto Mangunkusumo National General Hospital, Jakarta, Indonesia, and written informed consent, four American Society of Anesthesiologists (ASA) Grade I, II and III patients undergoing PCNL were recruited to the study. Exclusion criteria included morbid obesity, single functional kidney, contraindications to regional anaesthesia and pregnancy.

Prior to the surgery, the patients' vital signs were recorded. Supplementation of three litres per minute oxygen using a nasal cannula was used until the surgery was completed. Intravenous propofol was used on all subjects to attain moderate-grade sedation (Ramsay Sedation Scale 4).

ESP was done under ultrasound guidance using a linear transducer 6-13 MHz. The block site was performed on the same side as the PCNL using an ultrasound placed on paramedian/longitudinal position at the T9 level to identify its spinous processes. Erector spinae muscles superficial to the processes were identified. Afterward, local infiltration anaesthesia was administered into the skin with 3 mL of 2% lidocaine. Following the local infiltration, the block was performed using a 22G insulated needle 100 mm in length with an in-plane approach from cranial to caudal until the tip of the needle touched the cranial side of the T9 spinous processes. Normal saline solution was used to confirm the needle tip position. After fluid distribution to the cranial and caudal sides was observed, 25 mL of 0.5% isobaric bupivacaine mixed with 1:200,000 epinephrine was injected in aliquots of 5 ml until breathing signs (the separation of erector spinae muscles from transversal processes) were observed.

Before urethral manipulation, patients were given fentanyl 50 mcg intravenously. Sedation was maintained throughout the procedure. Following injection, vital signs and signs of local anaesthetic toxicity were carefully observed until the surgery was completed. Thirty minutes after injection, skin clamping was performed to determine the effectiveness of the ESP block. If no movement or change in vital signs occurred following clamping, the ESP block was deemed effective. However, if there were movements or vital sign changes (more than 30% from the baseline) during the surgery and intravenous propofol had reached 3.5 mcg/mL, conversion to general anaesthesia was planned.

The PCNL surgical procedure was carried out according to standard protocol. Operative time, intraoperative events, hospital stay duration and complications were recorded for each subject.

After the surgery, 1 gram of intravenous paracetamol was administered every eight hours to manage postoperative pain. However, if the pain persisted, a rescue dose of tramadol 50 mg intravenously was administered according to the numeric rating score (NRS). Postoperatively, patients were assessed for pain using NRS at rest and during movement. Patient-controlled analgesia (PCA) tramadol was provided for the patient and started when the patient arrived in the ward.

Results

The ESP block technique was successful in all four patients at the first attempt. No patient experienced problems during injection of the anaesthetic solution or insertion of the needle. Table 1 presents the characteristics of the subjects in this chapter.

Table 1. Characteristics of Subjects

Characteristics	Patient 1	Patient 2	Patient 3	Patient 4
Age (years)	47	39	47	48
Sex	Male	Male	Female	Male
ASA grade	3	3	2	1
PCNL side	Left	Left	Right	Right
Renal calculi size (mm)	37x17x15	24x18x19	11x11x9	15x12x11
Duration of surgery (min)	90	150	110	95
Comorbidities	Acute kidney injury	Chronic kidney disease, hypertension, anaemia	Hypokalaemia	None

An effective sensory block was achieved within 30 minutes for every patient. Following the block injection, cardiovascular changes were minimal. Hemodynamic stability was achieved in all subjects. However, one patient had to be converted to general anaesthesia due to excessive movement requiring deeper sedation at 60 minutes following the incision.

All surgeries were completed in less than 120 minutes, except for Patient 2. The NRS score for all patients peaked at six hours postoperatively. Most patients experienced pain with a numeric rating score of < 5 in the first 24 hours post-ESP block. All postoperative pain cases were treated with intravenous tramadol administration using PCA, which started immediately when the patient arrived in the ward. Table 3 presents the results of the anaesthesia.

Table 2. Intraoperative vital signs

Vital Signs	Baseline				*15 min*				*30 min*			
	BP	HR	RR	O_2	BP	HR	RR	O_2	BP	HR	RR	O_2
Patient 1	110/70	68	28	99	94/57	54	11	99	101/64	57	14	99
Patient 2	162/125	84	12	99	135/85	80	11	99	130/80	65	12	99
Patient 3	134/83	66	22	99	105/63	58	20	99	126/73	49	20	99
Patient 4	140/91	89	17	99	172/109	89	17	99	144/89	74	20	99

Vital Signs	*45 min*				*60 min*			
	BP	HR	RR	O_2	BP	HR	RR	O_2
Patient 1	112/64	61	13	99	132/72	56	16	99
Patient 2	160/104	62	13	99	168/100	70	13	99
Patient 3	106/68	54	16	99	97/64	55	16	99
Patient 4	146/97	68	15	99	150/94	74	23	99

Vital Signs	*75 min*				*90 min*				*105 min*			
	BP	HR	RR	O_2	BP	HR	RR	O_2	BP	HR	RR	O_2
Patient 1	100/65	60	18	99	105/60	65	16	99	106/63	61	17	99
Patient 2	163/106	69	12	99	161/118	71	11	99	162/122	65	12	99
Patient 3	108/73	63	16	99	111/75	48	16	99	101/74	50	21	99
Patient 4	140/87	70	23	99	141/93	64	24	99				

Vital Signs	*120 min*				*Recovery Room*			
	BP	HR	RR	O_2	BP	HR	RR	O_2
Patient 1					111/74	68	18	99
Patient 2	170/130	66	12	19	157/109	77	14	98
Patient 3					128/102	56	20	99
Patient 4					140/90	97	20	99

BP: blood pressure (mmHg), HR: heart rate (beats per minute), RR: respiration rate (rate per minute), O_2: oxygen saturation (percentage)

Table 3. Anaesthetic outcomes

Characteristics	Patient 1	Patient 2	Patient 3	Patient 4
Pain on skin clamping	No	No	No	No
Conversion to general anaesthesia	No	Yes	No	No
NRS score				
At recovery room	0	0	2	5
6 hours postoperative	1	7	3	4
12 hours postoperative	0	5	1	2
18 hours postoperative	0	5	1	2
24 hours postoperative	0	5	3	1
Additional tramadol (mg)	None	150	30	70
Postoperative length of stay (days)	4	5	2	4
Postoperative complication	None	Nausea	None	None

After the surgery, the patients were treated in the ward for 2-7 days before being discharged. Only one patient experienced nausea as a postoperative complication, which was treated with oral medication. There were no reported complications of haemothorax or hematoma.

Discussion

ESP block is an effective technique for managing neuropathic pain following pain after thoracic surgery, metastasis or malunion of ribs [3]. This technique deposits local anaesthetic into a plane between the two fascial layers (most anterior layer and deepest layer of the erector spinae muscle) and the tip of the transverse process, allowing local anaesthetic to spread to the craniocaudal side, paravertebral space and epidural space. This technique enables us to block the pain and sympathetic fibres with only a small amount of local anaesthetic. One of the advantages of the ESP block is its enormous level of safety due to its needle insertion site, which is relatively far from the nerves, great vessels, epidural space and pleura.

The use of ultrasound contributes immensely to the success of ESP blocks. Previous studies have shown that the ultrasound-guided nerve block is associated with a greater overall success rate [4]. As it is used to better visualise the structures around the injection site, ultrasound use may reduce the risk of infection, pneumothorax or even failed ESP block. Our study demonstrates a similar finding.

Few studies have discussed the use of ESP block as an anaesthetic technique in surgical procedures. Kimachi et al. reported a case-control study in which ESP block was effectively used as the sole anaesthetic for a unilateral mastectomy with axillary dissection performed in a patient at high risk for cardiovascular complications. Good results and minimal side effects were obtained in this study [5]. A prospective study from Malawat et al. showed that the average time to achieve complete surgical anaesthesia following ESP block was 31.5 minutes and the average time to administer first postoperative analgesia was 41.73 hours [6]. Therefore, we waited for about 30 minutes to ensure that the onset had been achieved in this chapter.

Successful surgical anaesthesia during PCNL is determined when a technique can block sensory and visceral pain during painful procedures without additional nerve blocks. This includes several stages of PCNL, including skin incision for tract dilatation, intracorporeal lithotripsy and evacuation of the stone fragment.4 In our study, success was established by performing skin clamping before the incision and observing movements or significant vital signs changes throughout the procedure. In line with other studies, stable vital signs were determined as changes in blood pressure and a heart rate less than 20% of the baseline value [7, 8] All of our patients showed no movement or vital sign changes of more than 20% in response to the skin clamping, which showed that ESP blocks at the level of T9 (lower thoracic level) were sufficient to block somatic and visceral pain originating from T7-L2, which are needed for the PCNL procedure (abdominal pelvic surgery) [9].

Hemodynamic stability in ESP blocks was maintained better than in other regional anaesthetic techniques. Although local anaesthetic drugs are spread into the epidural space, this phenomenon does not show significant sympathectomy and hypotension effects [10]. In our study, it was delivered with no significant hypotension encountered in all patients. However, one patient who had no response during skin clamping had to be converted to general anaesthesia due to excessive movement following TCI propofol concentration of 3.5mcg/ml. The phenomenon might have been caused by inconsistent spreading of the ESP block local anaesthetic.

To minimise local anaesthesia toxicity due to the high volume given to each patient, we calculated the maximum dosage of bupivacaine before the injection (< 3 mg/kg) and added epinephrine to rule out intravascular injection. In our study, no local anaesthesia toxicity developed.

Kamal et al. reported that the total tramadol consumption 24 hours after spinal anaesthesia for PCNL procedures reached an average of 125 mg. This finding showed that postoperative pain scores and the need for opioids are still high in the PCNL procedure after administering general and regional anesthesia [11]. In our study, almost all subjects needed intravenously administered tramadol postoperatively. However, most subjects only needed a small dose of tramadol to treat the pain (< 125 mg tramadol in 24 hours). Therefore, it can be concluded that ESP block can provide sufficient analgesia for up to 24 hours postoperatively.

The limitation of this chapter is its small sample size treated in a single health centre, which limits the generalisation of this chapter's findings. Furthermore, the nature of ESP, which is highly operator dependent, may hinder its applicability in centres without any trained operator.

Conclusion

ESP block is a feasible alternative for providing surgical anaesthesia in patients undergoing PCNL. However, further studies are needed to measure its applicability in all PCNL procedures.

Competing Interests

The authors declare that there is no conflict of interest in this chapter.

Acknowledgments

This article was presented in the 6th International Conference and Exhibition on Indonesian Medical Education and Research Institute (6th ICE on IMERI), Faculty of Medicine, Universitas Indonesia. We thank the 6th ICE on IMERI committee, who had supported the peer-review and manuscript preparation for publication to Nova Science Publishers, Inc.

References

[1] Astram, A., N. Rasyid, P. Birowo, P. Pryambodho, and C. Susilo. Success of percutaneous nephrolithotomy: Comparing spinal anesthesia with general anesthesia. *Indones. J. Urol.* 2015;1:106–206.

[2] Zanetti S P, Talso M, Palmisano F, Longo F, Gallioli A, Fontana M, De Lorenzis E, Sampogna G, Boeri L, Albo G, Trinchieri A, Montanari E. Comparison among the available stone treatment techniques from the first European Association of Urology Section of Urolithiasis (EULIS) Survey: Do we have a Queen? *PLoS One.* 2018 Nov 2;13(11):e0205159. doi: 10.1371/journal.pone.0205159.

[3] Peng P, Finlayson R, Lee S H, Bhatia A [eds.]. Ultrasound for interventional pain management: *An illustrated procedural guide.* Cham: Springer;2020. 61–62 p.

[4] Gelfand H J, Ouanes J P, Lesley M R, Ko P S, Murphy J D, Sumida S M, Isaac G R, Kumar K, Wu C L. Analgesic efficacy of ultrasound-guided regional anesthesia: a meta-analysis. *J Clin Anesth.* 2011 Mar;23(2):90-6. doi: 10.1016/j.jclinane. 2010.12.005.

[5] Kimachi P P, Martins E G, Peng P, Forero M. The erector spinae plane block provides complete surgical anesthesia in breast surgery: A case report. *A A Pract.* 2018 Oct 1;11(7):186-188. doi: 10.1213/XAA.0000000000000777.

[6] Malawat A, Verma K, Jethava D, Jethava D D. Erector spinae plane block for complete surgical anaesthesia and postoperative analgesia for breast surgeries: A prospective feasibility study of 30 cases. *Indian J. Anaesth.* 2020 Feb;64(2):118-124. doi: 10.4103/ija.IJA_639_19.

[7] Yoon J Y, Park C G, Kim E J, Choi B M, Yoon J U, Kim Y H, Lee M O, Han K S, Ahn J H. Optimal effect-site concentration of remifentanil to prevent hemodynamic changes during nasotracheal intubation using a video laryngoscope. *J. Dent. Anesth. Pain Med.* 2020 Aug;20(4):195-202. doi: 10.17245/jdapm.2020.20.4.195.

[8] Kim W S, Byeon G J, Song B J, Lee H J. Availability of preoperative anxiety scale as a predictive factor for hemodynamic changes during induction of anesthesia. *Korean J. Anesthesiol.* 2010 Apr;58(4):328-33. doi: 10.4097/kjae.2010.58.4.328.

[9] Singh S, Ranjan R, Lalin D. A new indication of erector spinae plane block for perioperative analgesia is total hip replacement surgery - A case report. *Indian J. Anaesth.* 2019 Apr;63(4):310-311. doi: 10.4103/ija.IJA_25_19.

[10] Krishna S N, Chauhan S, Bhoi D, Kaushal B, Hasija S, Sangdup T, Bisoi A K. Bilateral erector spinae plane block for acute post-surgical pain in adult cardiac surgical patients: A randomized controlled trial. *J Cardiothorac. Vasc. Anesth.* 2019 Feb;33(2):368-375. doi: 10.1053/j.jvca.2018.05.050.

[11] Kamal M, Sharma P, Singariya G, Jain R. Feasibility and complications of spinal anaesthesia in percutaneous nephrolithotomy: Our experience. *J. Clin. Diagn. Res.* 2017 Jun;11(6):UC08-UC11. doi: 10.7860/JCDR/2017/26425.10111.

Chapter 11

Impact of Diaphragm Excursion Ultrasound in Predicting the Duration of Mechanical Ventilation: A Case Series

Anung Darmawan[1,*], Indro Mulyono[1,2] and Andi Ade Wijaya[1]

[1]Departement of Anesthesiology and Intensive Care, Faculty of Medicine, Universitas Indonesia, Jakarta, Indonesia

[2]Intensive Care Unit, Cipto Mangunkusumo Hospital, Jakarta, Indonesia

Abstract

The diaphragm is the primary muscle used for inspiration in spontaneous breathing. Patients who failed a spontaneous breathing from any causes usually need mechanical ventilation until the cause of the failure is resolved. Mechanical ventilation has side effects, such as ventilator-induced diaphragm dysfunction (VIDD), which is associated with prolonged mechanical ventilation and weaning failure. An assessment of diaphragm function, such as diaphragm excursion or diaphragm movement using ultrasonography, is chosen because the procedure is safe, non-invasive, has no radiation and is easy to use at bedside, but this is not yet a routine procedure. In the M mode of ultrasonography, the diaphragmatic excursion (displacement, mm) is measured with a cut-off limit above 10 mm and an important clinical finding in predicting successful weaning from mechanical ventilation. This chapter is a case series with subjects who were patients with a primary diagnosis of respiratory failure on mechanical ventilation in the ICU. Diaphragm excursion was documented when the patients were being weaned from

[*] Corresponding Author's Email: anung.darmawan@yahoo.com.

In: The 6th Annual International Conference …
Editors: M. Maidarti, H. Winarto, C. O. M. Jasirwan et al.
ISBN: 978-1-68507-925-3

mechanical ventilation. A diaphragm excursion > 10 mm was counted as normal, while a diaphragm excursion < 10 mm was low. The duration of mechanical ventilation was also documented. During the study period, 10 patients were documented. Five of those subjects had normal diaphragm excursions and had received mechanical ventilation for fewer than seven days. The other five subjects had low diaphragm excursion and had received mechanical ventilation for more than seven days. In conclusion, diaphragm excursion using ultrasonography has an impact on the duration of mechanical ventilation.

Keywords: diaphragm excursion, duration of mechanical ventilation

Case Series

Introduction

The diaphragm is a dome-shaped muscle that splits the intrathoracic space and intraabdominal space. As the main respiratory muscle, the diaphragm has nerve innervation from the phrenic nerve from the C3 to C5 nerve roots. When the diaphragm contracts, the intraabdominal space is pushed down, and the intraabdominal pressure increases in the apposition zone. Then, the ribcage expands and increases the intrathoracic space. Illness that disrupts diaphragm innervation, contractility or ribcage expansion can cause diaphragm dysfunction [1].

The use of a mechanical ventilator that disturbs respiratory muscle dysfunction is called ventilator-induced diaphragm dysfunction (VIDD). Diaphragm dysfunction commonly occurs in mechanically ventilated patients, but the diaphragm has an important role in successful weaning from mechanical ventilation.

Diaphragm visualisation using ultrasonography sound has been practiced for more than 40 years. New technology in ultrasound has made assessment of diaphragm function and size while using mechanical ventilation feasible. There are two assessments of diaphragm function: diaphragm excursion (DE) and diaphragm thickness. Diaphragm excursion is assessed by counting the distance of the diaphragm muscle while respirating [2]. Diaphragm excursion is assessed by placing a probe array in the subcostal margin of the midclavicular line to examine the 1/3 posterior part of the diaphragm. Although some research has used the B mode (produce a two-dimensional image of the underlying tissue) to assess the diaphragm, the M mode (or motion mode produce time motion display of the ultrasound wave along a chosen ultrasound line) can also visualise diaphragm movement in real time and can measure diaphragm movement accurately [3].

Although this ultrasonography examination function of the diaphragm is not common in the ICU, ultrasonography has benefits such as being simple, non-invasive and without radiation. It can also be performed at the patient's bedside and can be used for clinical and research findings.

Objectives

This chapter assesses diaphragmatic excursion using ultrasonography and its outcome on the duration of mechanical ventilation.

Materials and Methods

In this chapter, we conduct research on patients using mechanical ventilation in the ICU in the emergency room and the ICU in the adult room from November to December 2020. The diaphragm excursion was measured using ultrasonography in the M mode with a 3.5-5 MHz probe. The probe was placed in the space between the 8th to 10th ribs on the midaxillary line. The diaphragm excursion was documented when the patients were being weaned from mechanical ventilation. A diaphragm excursion > 10 mm is normal, while a diaphragm excursion < 10 mm is low. The duration of mechanical ventilation was also documented.

Results

In this chapter of the 10 patients, there were five cases with low diaphragm excursion (DE < 10 mm) and prolonged duration of mechanical ventilation (> 7 days). The other five cases had normal diaphragm excursion (DE > 10 mm) and had received mechanical ventilation for fewer than seven days.

Table 1. Patients' characteristics

Case	Baseline of Patient						
	Age (years old)	Weight (kg)	Height (cm)	BMI	Blood Pressure (mmHg)	Heart Rate (beat/minute)	GCS (Eye Movement Verbal)
1	35	40	150	17.8	90/60	120	E1 M3 Vett
2	26	56	160	21.9	140/76	118	E4 M6 Vett
3	20	65	169	22.8	97/45	130	E4 M6 Vett
4	56	53	160	20.7	131/70	108	E4 M6 Vett
5	57	55	160	21.5	100/60	100	E4 M6 Vett
6	17	75	175	24.5	120/75	120	E4 M6 Vett
7	20	60	160	23.4	130/71	115	E2 M5 Vett
8	22	53	155	22.1	100/60	80	E4 M6 Vett
9	53	73	170	25.3	63/47	91	E3 M6 Vett
10	69	65	165	23.9	140/90	96	E4 M6 Vett

Table 2. Results

Case	Cause of Patient's Mechanical Ventilation Need	Diaphragm Excursion (mm)	Duration on Mechanical Ventilation (days)	Patients Outcome
1	ARDS, SLE	7.7	> 7	Difficult weaning
2	After caesarean section surgery	14.3	< 7	Simple weaning
3	After limb salvage surgery	14.5	< 7	Simple weaning
4	After laparotomy surgery	7.6	> 7	Difficult weaning
5	After debridement, Sepsis	9.4	> 7	Difficult weaning
6	After laparotomy surgery	21.4	< 7	Simple weaning
7	Sub arachnoid haemorrhage	8.8	> 7	Difficult weaning
8	After flap fibula surgery	15.1	< 7	Simple weaning
9	ARDS, CKD	5.8	> 7	Difficult weaning
10	Sepsis	18.9	< 7	Simple weaning

Discussion

Weaning failure could lead to prolonged mechanical ventilation and duration of hospitalisation in the ICU [2]. However, delayed weaning could lead to risks from mechanical ventilation, such as barotrauma, ventilator-associated pneumonia and ventilator-induced diaphragmatic atrophy [2]. Therefore, patients need to be weaned as soon as possible from mechanical ventilation to prevent diaphragm dysfunction and infection and to lower the duration of ICU hospitalisation [2].

Many things, including sepsis, electrolyte imbalance, hyperinflation and critical illness (e.g., polyneuropathy), could cause diaphragm dysfunction in ICU patients. Patients could have diaphragm dysfunction since the first day they are admitted to the ICU and intubated [4].

Diaphragm excursion measurements have been performed since ultrasonography has been available in the ICU. A normal Diaphragm Excursion would make the weaning process easier and reduce the duration of ventilation. There are some cut-offs in the Diaphragm Excursion measurement. We used 10 mm as a cut-off for normal diaphragm excursion. An increase in Diaphragm Excursion means an increase in diaphragm distance when breathing, which means better movement of the diaphragm [5].

Of the 10 patients in our study, five had received mechanical ventilation for fewer than seven days with normal diaphragm excursion, (Diaphragm Excursion > 10 mm) showing that monitoring diaphragm excursion assessed by ultrasonography can be used as an important factor in predicting the duration of mechanical ventilation.

A study by Osman also found that examining diaphragm function by ultrasonography is a quick and non-invasive method in the weaning process that has high accuracy and can be used as a predicting factor of the weaning process in critically ill patients [5, 6].

Conclusion

In this case series, we found that diaphragm excursion assessment by ultrasonography can be used in predicting the duration of mechanical ventilation in critically ill ICU patients.

Competing Interests

The authors state that there is no conflict of interest.

Acknowledgments

This article was presented in the 6th International Conference and Exhibition on Indonesian Medical Education and Research Institute (6th ICE on IMERI), Faculty of Medicine, Universitas Indonesia. We thank the 6th ICE on IMERI committee, who had supported the peer-review and manuscript preparation for publication to Nova Science Publishers, Inc.

References

[1] McCool F D, Tzelepis GE. Dysfunction of the diaphragm. *N. Engl. J. Med.* 2012 Mar 8;366(10):932-42. doi: 10.1056/NEJMra1007236.

[2] Li C, Li X, Han H, Cui H, Wang G, Wang Z. Diaphragmatic ultrasonography for predicting ventilator weaning: A meta-analysis. *Medicine (Baltimore).* 2018 Jun;97(22):e10968. doi: 10.1097/MD.0000000000010968.

[3] Turton P, ALAidarous S, Welters I. A narrative review of diaphragm ultrasound to predict weaning from mechanical ventilation: where are we and where are we heading? *Ultrasound J.* 2019 Feb 28;11(1):2. doi: 10.1186/s13089-019-0117-8.

[4] Sigala I, Vassilakopoulos T. Diaphragmatic ultrasound as a monitoring tool in the intensive care unit. *Ann. Transl. Med.* 2017 Feb;5(4):79. doi: 10.21037/atm.2017.01.68.

[5] Osman A M, Hashim R M. Diaphragmatic and lung ultrasound application as new predictive indices for the weaning process in ICU patients. *Egypt. J. Radiol. Nucl. Med.*. 2017; 48(1):61–66. doi: 10.1016/j.ejrnm.2017.01.005.

[6] Arshad H, Khan A, Khalil A, and Ashgar A. Diaphragmatic excursion: does it predict successful weaning from mechanical ventilation? *J. Coll. Physicians Surg. Pak.* 2017;27(12):743–46.

Chapter 12

Using the Ultrasound Diaphragm Thickening Fraction to Predict the Length of Ventilator Use: A Case Series

Rudy Nugroho[1,*] and Indro Mulyono[1,2]

[1]Departement of Anesthesiology and Intensive Care, Faculty of Medicine, Universitas Indonesia, Jakarta, Indonesia

[2]Intensive Care Unit, Cipto Mangunkusumo Hospital, Jakarta, Indonesia

Abstract

Background: Ventilators are often used in the management of critically ill patients. The diaphragm is the primary muscle used for inspiration, and a diaphragm ultrasound can be used to assess diaphragmatic muscle dysfunction. Decreased diaphragmatic muscle thickness is an important component of diaphragmatic dysfunction, resulting in difficulty being weaned off ventilators. The uniqueness of this case series was using the diaphragm thickening fraction based on ultrasound, which is a safe, non-invasive procedure that can be performed bedside to predict the length of ventilator use.

Case Presentation: In this case series, we observed 10 patients with a main diagnosis of respiratory failure who were treated using ventilators. Examination of the diaphragm thickening fraction was carried out within 24 hours of the patient using a ventilator. Patients were treated with usual standard care, and the length of time on ventilator was recorded.

Management and Outcome: Of the 10 patients observed, five had a diaphragm thickening fraction < 30% and five had a diaphragm thickening fraction > 30%. The five patients with diaphragm thickening fraction < 30% were on a ventilator for more than seven days, whereas

[*] Corresponding Author's Email: ruudnugroho@gmail.com.

In: The 6th Annual International Conference …
Editors: M. Maidarti, H. Winarto, C. O. M. Jasirwan et al.
ISBN: 978-1-68507-925-3

those with a diaphragm thickening fraction > 30% used a ventilator for less than seven days.

Conclusion: The diaphragm thickening fraction can help to predict the length of ventilator use, with a cut-off of 30%.

Keywords: diaphragm thickening fraction, length of ventilator use

Case Series

Introduction

Weaning from mechanical ventilation is essential in treating critically intubated patients and receiving mechanical ventilation. Weaning from mechanical ventilation accounts for about 40% of the duration of mechanical ventilation. Although most of the weaning process is easy, 20-25% of patients have difficulty being weaned from mechanical ventilation [1]. Under normal circumstances, the diaphragm muscle is the main muscle during inspiration, whereas expiration is a passive movement, governed by the relaxation of the inspiratory muscles [2]. To facilitate early detection of respiratory muscle weakness, a measurement or examination method is needed that can be carried out in the ICU, is easy to perform, non-invasive and repeatable. Examinations using ultrasound are growing because of its ability to assess various aspects of muscles, it can be performed directly beside the patient (bedside) and it is relatively cheaper than other imaging examination modalities [3].

Ultrasonography can be used to assess diaphragmatic muscle dysfunction to predict failure in the mechanical ventilation weaning process, assess the respiratory workload and measure the progression of diaphragmatic muscle atrophy. Decreased diaphragmatic muscle mass thickness is an important component of diaphragmatic dysfunction, resulting in difficulty being weaned from mechanical ventilation [4]. The diaphragm thickening fraction is assessed by measuring the thickness of the diaphragm muscle during expiration and subtracting it from the thickness of the diaphragm muscle during inspiration, dividing it by the thickness of the diaphragm muscle during expiration and multiplying it by 100%. Several studies have provided the best minimal diaphragm thickening fraction for predicting successful extubation [5-8].

Although most studies [5-8] have shown that diaphragm thickening fraction can predict successful extubation, there are no studies showing that the diaphragm thickening fraction can predict the length of ventilator use. This case series describes the phenomenon of diaphragm thickening fraction using ultrasound, which is a safe, non-invasive procedure that can be performed bedside to predict the length of ventilator use. Estimating the length of time on a ventilator can help to estimate the length of stay, the cost of treatment and the prognosis of the patient's recovery.

Materials and Methods

In this case series, we observed 10 patients with main diagnosis respiratory failure who were treated using ventilators in Cipto Mangunkusumo Hospital from October until December 2020. Examination of the ultrasound diaphragm thickening fraction was carried out within 24 hours of the patient using a ventilator. Sequential organ failure assessment (SOFA) scores and PaO2/FiO2 ratio of patients were also recorded in the first 24 hours. All examinations were carried out in the morning. Patients were treated with usual standard care, and the length of time on ventilator was recorded. An extensive literature search was conducted through Medline/PubMed and Google Scholar using the search terms 'weaning' OR 'ventilator' OR 'diaphragm ultrasound' OR 'diaphragm thickening fraction' to identify relevant articles.

Results

We examined 10 patients who were treated with ventilators in Cipto Mangunkusumo Hospital from October to December 2020. All the cases were aged 17-70 years with an initial diagnosis of pneumonia and the baseline characteristics shown in Table 1. SOFA scores for predicting organ dysfunction varied between 4 and 11. All patients had a P/F ratio between 200 and 300 (Table 2).

Discussion

In this case series, we found that diaphragmatic muscle dysfunction was a common occurrence during ICU admission. Under normal circumstances, the diaphragm muscle is the main muscle used during inspiration, whereas expiration is a passive movement, which is governed by the relaxation of the inspiratory muscles. Respiratory muscle weakness in critically ill patients is associated with increased duration of ventilator use and increased patient return to the ICU [2]. To facilitate the early detection of respiratory muscle weakness, a measurement or examination method is needed that can be carried out in the ICU, is easy to perform, non-invasive and can be repeated. Examinations using ultrasound are growing because of its ability to assess various aspects of muscles and it can be performed bedside [3].

Table 1. Baseline Characteristics of the Patients

Case	Age (years)	Height (cm)	Weight (kg)	BMI (kg/m2)	Blood pressure (mmHg)	Heart Rate (x/minute)	Temp (°C)
1	35	162	64	24.42	104/61	124	36.7
2	20	151	63	27.63	126/71	100	37.1
3	36	161	55	21.23	113/54	92	36.2
4	62	161	68	26.25	97/65	135	37.3
5	59	152	65	28.13	101/59	112	36.8
6	43	150	59	26.22	135/76	93	36.9
7	25	145	57	27.14	129/63	104	37.0
8	57	158	65	26.10	104/62	109	36.6
9	37	158	62	24.89	127/54	110	36.2
10	53	156	75	30.86	164/83	127	37.3

Table 2. Clinical findings of patients

Case	Age (years)	SOFA Score	P/F Ratio	DTF (%)	Length of Time on Ventilator (days)
1	35	11	226	15.4	10
2	20	5	289	43	2
3	36	4	259	36.3	3
4	62	10	277	26.2	9
5	59	9	202	29.6	12
6	43	5	279	46.7	4
7	25	4	292	32.4	3
8	57	10	237	20.4	9
9	37	5	274	35.3	6
10	53	11	221	16.4	10

SOFA = Sequential Organ Failure Assessment; DTF = Diaphragm Thickening Fraction; P/F ratio = PaO_2/FiO_2 ratio.

Diaphragmatic muscle dysfunction, which can be caused by various factors such as comorbid disease, neuromuscular disorders and trauma, can make it difficult to wean patients from mechanical ventilation. As the main inspiratory muscle, the diaphragm can become dysfunctional due to various lung diseases as well as the use of positive pressure from mechanical ventilation [9]. Ultrasound examinations can be used to assess the dysfunction of the diaphragm muscle to predict failure in the mechanical ventilation weaning process, assess the workload of respiration and determine the progress of diaphragmatic muscle atrophy [10]. Decreased diaphragmatic muscle mass thickness is an important component of diaphragmatic dysfunction resulting in difficulty in weaning mechanical ventilation [4].

Several studies have shown that diaphragmatic ultrasonography can predict the success of weaning from mechanical ventilation. Several recent studies have indicated that the threshold value for predicting successful extubation or weaning failure is 30-36% in the diaphragm thickening fraction as the most sensitive and specific value [11].

In our case series, of the 10 patients examined, 5 had a diaphragmatic thickening fraction < 30% and 5 had a diaphragmatic thickening fraction > 30%. Patients with diaphragmatic thickening fraction < 30% used the ventilator for 9-12 days, whereas patients with a diaphragm thickening fraction > 30% used the ventilator for 2-6 days. The findings of this case series show that patients with a low diaphragm thickening fraction can use a ventilator for more than 7 days, whereas patients with a high diaphragm thickening fraction can use a ventilator for less than 7 days. The SOFA scores in these patients were quite variable, but the P/F Ratio of these patients was sufficiently uniform to reduce the possibility of bias.

Ferrari et al., reported that the diaphragmatic thickening fraction could predict weaning after a spontaneous breathing trial. This study suggests that a diaphragmatic thickening fraction value > 36% is associated with successful weaning.12 Samanta et al., stated that the diaphragm thickening fraction can predict simple weaning; that is, patients can be extubated on their first spontaneous breathing trial without difficulty. A diaphragmatic thickening fraction value > 26% can predict easy weaning of mechanical ventilation with a sensitivity of 97% and a specificity of 81%.5 Although these two studies used the diaphragm thickening fraction for successful extubation, this case series examines the possibility of using the diaphragm thickening fraction to predict the length of ventilator use.

Conclusion

In this case series, diaphragmatic muscle dysfunction on ICU admission was found to be common. Ultrasound examination of the diaphragm thickening fraction can help predict the duration of ventilator use. These findings strengthen the utility of diaphragmatic ultrasonography, which is easy to perform, non-invasive and can be performed directly beside the patient.

Competing Interests

The authors state that there is no conflict of interest.

Acknowledgments

This article was presented in the 6th International Conference and Exhibition on Indonesian Medical Education and Research Institute (6th ICE on IMERI), Faculty of Medicine, Universitas Indonesia. We thank the 6th ICE on IMERI committee, who had supported the peer-review and manuscript preparation for publication to Nova Science Publishers, Inc.

References

[1] Boles J M, Bion J, Connors A, Herridge M, Marsh B, Melot C, Pearl R, Silverman H, Stanchina M, Vieillard-Baron A, Welte T. Weaning from mechanical ventilation. *Eur. Respir. J.* 2007 May;29(5):1033-56. doi: 10.1183/09031936.00010206.

[2] Jonkman A H, Jansen D, Heunks L M. Novel insights in ICU-acquired respiratory muscle dysfunction: implications for clinical care. *Crit. Care*. 2017 Mar 21;21(1):64. doi: 10.1186/s13054-017-1642-0.

[3] Latronico N, Herridge M, Hopkins R O, Angus D, Hart N, Hermans G, Iwashyna T, Arabi Y, Citerio G, Ely E W, Hall J, Mehta S, Puntillo K, Van den Hoeven J, Wunsch H, Cook D, Dos Santos C, Rubenfeld G, Vincent J L, Van den Berghe G, Azoulay E, Needham D M. The ICM research agenda on intensive care unit-acquired weakness. *Intensive Care Med.* 2017 Sep;43(9):1270-1281. doi: 10.1007/s00134-017-4757-5.

[4] Zambon M, Greco M, Bocchino S, Cabrini L, Beccaria P F, Zangrillo A. Assessment of diaphragmatic dysfunction in the critically ill patient with ultrasound: a systematic review. *Intensive Care Med.* 2017 Jan;43(1):29-38. doi: 10.1007/s00134-016-4524-z.

[5] Samanta S, Singh R K, Baronia A K, Poddar B, Azim A, Gurjar M. Diaphragm thickening fraction to predict weaning-a prospective exploratory study. *J. Intensive Care*. 2017 Nov 13;5:62. doi: 10.1186/s40560-017-0258-4.

[6] Ferrari G, De Filippi G, Elia F, Panero F, Volpicelli G, Aprà F. Diaphragm ultrasound as a new index of discontinuation from mechanical ventilation. *Crit. Ultrasound J*. 2014 Jun 7;6(1):8. doi: 10.1186/2036-7902-6-8.

[7] Pirompanich P, Romsaiyut S. Use of diaphragm thickening fraction combined with rapid shallow breathing index for predicting success of weaning from mechanical ventilator in medical patients. *J. Intensive Care*. 2018 Feb 2;6:6. doi: 10.1186/s40560-018-0277-9.

[8] DiNino E, Gartman E J, Sethi J M, McCool FD. Diaphragm ultrasound as a predictor of successful extubation from mechanical ventilation. *Thorax*. 2014 May;69(5):423-7. doi: 10.1136/thoraxjnl-2013-204111.

[9] Supinski G S, Morris P E, Dhar S, Callahan L A. Diaphragm Dysfunction in Critical Illness. *Chest*. 2018 Apr;153(4):1040-1051. doi: 10.1016/j.chest.2017.08.1157.

[10] Jorens P G, Schepens T. Ultrasound: a novel translational tool to study diaphragmatic dysfunction in critical illness. *Ann. Transl. Med*. 2016 Dec;4(24):515. doi: 10.21037/atm.2016.12.49.

[11] Turton P, ALAidarous S, Welters I. A narrative review of diaphragm ultrasound to predict weaning from mechanical ventilation: where are we and where are we heading? *Ultrasound J*. 2019 Feb 28;11(1):2. doi: 10.1186/s13089-019-0117-8. PMID: 31359260; PMCID: PMC6638615.

[12] Ferrari G, De Filippi G, Elia F, Panero F, Volpicelli G, Aprà F. Diaphragm ultrasound as a new index of discontinuation from mechanical ventilation. *Crit Ultrasound J*. 2014 Jun 7;6(1):8. doi: 10.1186/2036-7902-6-8.

Chapter 13

How Transorbital Electrical Stimulation and Orthoptic Exercise Improves Ophthalmoplegia, Ptosis and Diplopia in Miller Fisher Syndrome: A Case Report

Rakhmawati Diyana[1,*], Rahmad[1], Bethasiwi Purbasari[2], Muhammad Ridwan[1] and Dwi Indriani L.[1]

[1]Department of Physical Medicine and Rehabilitation, Faculty of Medicine, University of Brawijaya - Dr Saiful Anwar General Hospital, Malang, East Java, Indonesia
[2]Interdisciplinary Graduate School of Medicine and Veterinary Medicine, Miyazaki University, Miyazaki, Japan

Abstract

Miller Fisher Syndrome (MFS) is one of several types of Guillain Barre Syndrome (GBS) that is characterised by a triad: ophthalmoplegia, areflexia/hyporeflexia and ataxia. The application of electrical stimulation (ES) has proven to improve several ophthalmic diseases. Although ES is not yet widely used to treat ophthalmoplegia, several studies have shown its benefits in improving eye movement. We report a case of a 29-year-old man who presented with GBS with ophthalmoplegia, ptosis and diplopia sequels. The patient's deep tendon reflexes had decreased, but there were no signs of ataxia. The patient had been admitted for a month previously because of weakness in the extremities and respiratory distress due to GBS, which had improved after three plasma exchanges and corticosteroid treatments.

* Corresponding Author's Email: rakhmawatid@student.ub.ac.id.

In: The 6th Annual International Conference …
Editors: M. Maidarti, H. Winarto, C. O. M. Jasirwan et al.
ISBN: 978-1-68507-925-3

At a supporting examination, the patient had shown increased protein in a cerebrospinal fluid analysis and mild axonal motoric-sensory polyneuropathy in an electromyograph study. Anti-GQ1b immunoglobulin G was not evaluated. Transorbital ES and orthoptic exercises (OE) improve ophthalmoplegia, ptosis and diplopia sequels satisfyingly after five weeks of rehabilitation, allowing the patient to be functionally active in his work and daily activities.

Keywords: electrical stimulation, orthoptic exercise, ophthalmoplegia, diplopia, *Miller Fisher* Syndrome

Introduction

Miller Fisher Syndrome (MFS) is one of five types of Guillain Barre Syndrome (GBS) that is characterised by a triad: ophthalmoplegia, areflexia/hyporeflexia and ataxia [1, 2]. The pathophysiology is the cross-reaction of anti-ganglioside Q1b immunoglobulin G (anti-GQ1b IgG) that triggers the complement activation and macrophage infiltration that lead to the destruction of myelin, glia and axons, resulting in a disturbance in nerve conduction [1-3]. These antibodies are present in the serum of 85-90% of patients with MFS [3]. Although divided into several types, GBS can overlap from one type to another [4, 5].

Electrical stimulation (ES) is one treatment method that has been developed to improve ophthalmic diseases [4]. ES stimulates neurons along the visual pathway and enhances the production of neurotropic factors and growth factors that improve the symptoms of ophthalmic diseases [6, 7]. Studies on the application of ES for ophthalmoplegia are limited, but those that have been conducted show an improvement effect on ophthalmoplegia [8-10].

Among patients with GBS, overlapping with MFS symptoms is very rare and can have serious effects on patients, especially their quality of life, because weakness, shortness of breath, ophthalmoplegia and diplopia could interfere with patients' daily and working activities [7, 8]. Here, we report the case of a man with ophthalmoplegia, ptosis and diplopia preceded by weakness in the extremities and respiratory distress, who was diagnosed with GBS. The patient improved after a five-week rehabilitation programme involving transorbital ES and orthoptic exercises.

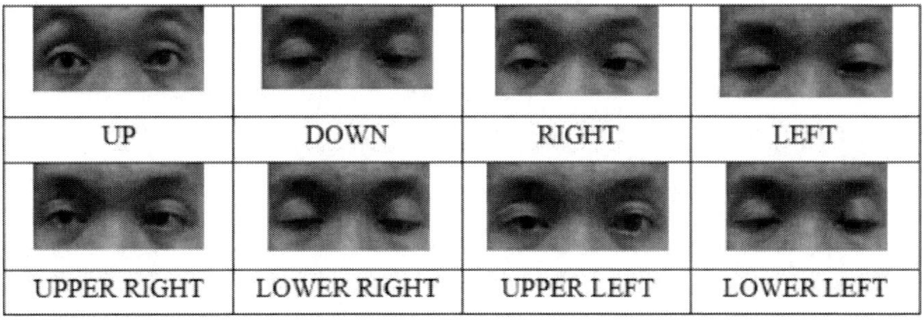

Figure 1. Ophthalmoplegia and ptosis at first visit to our PM&R Clinic.

Case Report

A 29-year-old man came to our Physical Medicine and Rehabilitation (PM&R) Outpatient Clinic and presented with ophthalmoplegia, ptosis and diplopia as sequels of GBS. This condition affected the patient's ability to identify the position, location and distance of the objects; reach, handle, and grasp objects; do his work as a florist; use gadgets; and drive.

A physical examination showed bilateral ophthalmoplegia and ptosis to the point that the patient could not fully open his eyes (Figure 1). The patient's pupil was isochoric, and the pupillary light reflexes and the corneal reflexes were normal. Subjectively, the patient said the visual distance of his diplopia was about 4 cm. The patient's deep tendon reflexes were decreased, but there were no signs of ataxia. The motoric strength of his extremities was improved but not fully recovered, with an average manual muscle testing (MMT) score of 4.

A month earlier, the patient had experienced diarrhoea and a common cold, but no fever. A week later, he developed weakness in the extremities and shortness of breath. He was admitted to Dr Saiful Anwar General Hospital, Malang, East Java, Indonesia, where he had three plasma exchanges and corticosteroids, but no ventilator was needed. The patient was discharged after four weeks of hospitalisation with improvements to extremity weakness and respiratory distress, but ophthalmoplegia, ptosis and diplopia remained. The patient was referred to the PM&R Outpatient Clinic at week 6 to receive treatment for the sequels.

At a supporting examination, the patient achieved positive results on the Nonne and Pandy test (normal range: negative), which indicated an increase in protein for the cerebrospinal fluid analysis. An electromyography study showed mild axonal motoric and sensory polyneuropathy. Anti-GQ1b IgG was not evaluated.

Specifically for ophthalmoplegia, ptosis and diplopia, we planned a rehabilitation programme using transorbital ES (Figure 2) at a bitemporal area with a frequency of 10 Hz, intensity of 5-10 mA and a duration of 15 minutes twice a week. The patient was also given orthoptic exercises (eye movement and eye-hand coordination) twice a week at the PM&R clinic, which he continued every day as home exercise programmes.

The patient routinely followed the five twice weekly (10 sessions) treatments as a rehabilitation programme. After completing the rehabilitation programme, the patient showed satisfactory improvements. The ophthalmoplegia was significantly improved (Figure 3), the ptosis was completely remitted and the subjective visual distance of diplopia was less than 1 cm (Figure 4). The patient could identify the position, location and distance of the objects; reach, handle, and grasp objects safely; return to his work as a florist; use gadgets; and drive. No adverse or unanticipated events were reported in this patient rehabilitation programme.

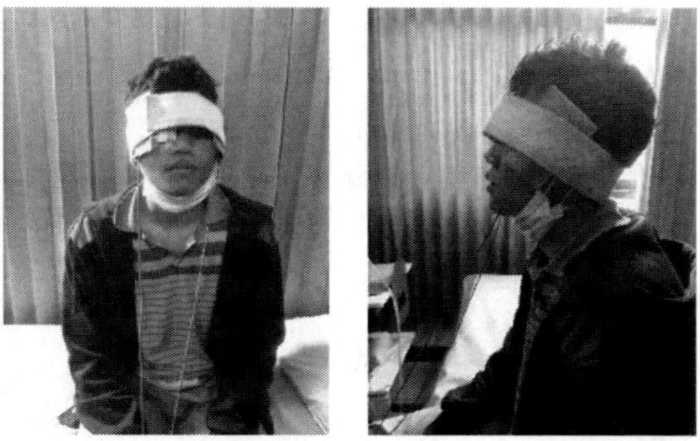

Figure 2. Transorbital ES.

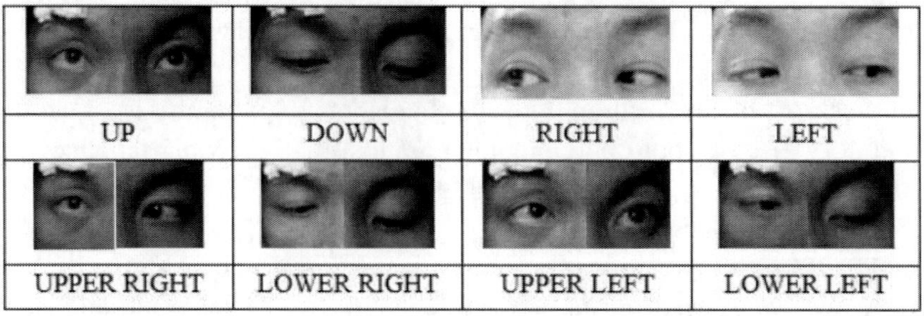

Figure 3. Ophthalmoplegia and ptosis after a five-week rehabilitation programme.

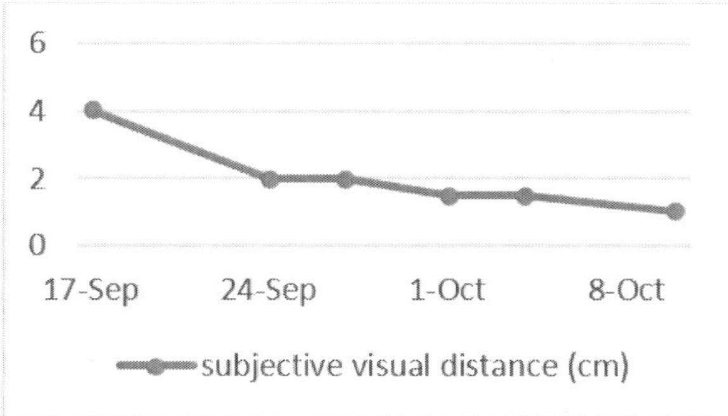

Figure 4. Patient's subjective visual distance of diplopia.

Discussion

ES for ophthalmic diseases can be applied in several ways: transorbital, transcorneal, transpalpebral, transchoroideal, epiretinal and subretinal [11]. Studies that have been conducted by applying ES to ophthalmic diseases have shown significant improvements in optic nerve lesion, optic neuropathy, retinopathy, macular degeneration, retinitis pigmentosa and amblyopia [11, 12]. Although ES is not widely used to treat ophthalmoplegia and its publications are very limited, several studies have shown its benefit in improving ophthalmoplegia and diplopia [13-15]. Arianda [13] and Putri et al. [15] described significant improvements in patients with ophthalmoplegia, ptosis and diplopia after administering ES and orthoptic exercises. Similarly, Liu et al. [14] described that electroacupuncture treatment improved eye movement and the quality of life of 12 patients with ophthalmoplegia, but the reports did not include patients with ophthalmoplegia caused by MFS.

The suggested mechanisms that are believed to underlie the effects of ES for ophthalmoplegia are that ES stimulates neurons along the visual pathway (including cranial nerves [oculomotor, trochlear and abducens] until the brainstem and its innervated muscles), increases the expression of neurotrophic factors, increases the expression of fibroblast growth factor, promotes neuronal survival by increasing intracellular Ca^{2+} influx and provides a neuroprotective effect that is significant in preventing secondary apoptosis [11, 12].

OE for ophthalmoplegia and diplopia can be done in several ways, including 'pencil push up,' accommodation-convergence bar, pen or dot convergence therapy, prism vergence exercises to build fusional vergence amplitudes, stereograms, the Brock string, the three-dot card and the high-tech option 'computerized orthoptic programmes' that are available for home use. Although the effects of OE on the paretic extraocular muscle and cranial nerve are still unknown, several studies have shown significant improvements in ophthalmoplegia and diplopia treated with OE. Possible mechanisms for the action of OE include the stimulation of axonal growth and/or remyelination through the release of trophic factors. Alternatively, OE may cause hypertrophy of existing intact neuro-muscular units [6, 10].

The limitation of this study is that it only reports on one case. The application of ES and orthoptic exercise is not widely used; hence, it is important to obtain more reports and research with bigger samples to ensure the effect of ES and orthoptic exercise.

Patients' Perspective

The patient had high motivation and completed the rehabilitation programme routinely. The patient was pleased with the treatment results because his vision improved. At the end of the treatment session, he could identify the position, location and distance of the objects; reach, handle, and grasp objects safely; return to his work as a florist; use gadgets; and drive. There were no adverse or unanticipated events reported.

Conclusion

The conclusion of this report is that transorbital ES and orthoptic exercise can improve ophthalmoplegia, ptosis and diplopia sequels of MFS; hence, patients can be functionally active in their work and daily activities and have a better quality of life.

Acknowledgments

This article was presented in the 6th International Conference and Exhibition on Indonesian Medical Education and Research Institute (6th ICE on IMERI), Faculty of Medicine, Universitas Indonesia. We thank the 6th ICE on IMERI committee, who had supported the peer-review and manuscript preparation for publication to Nova Science Publishers, Inc.

Competing Interests: The authors declare no conflicts of interest.

References

[1] Wijdicks EF, Klein CJ. Guillain-Barré Syndrome. *Mayo Clin. Proc.* 2017 Mar;92(3):467-479. doi: 10.1016/j.mayocp.2016.12.002.

[2] Al Othman B, Raabe J, Kini A, Lee AG. Update: the Miller Fisher variants of Guillain-Barré syndrome. *Curr. Opin. Ophthalmol.* 2019 Nov;30(6):462-466. doi: 10.1097/ICU.0000000000000611.

[3] Tsuzaki K, Tatsuno K, Inoue M, Tachibana N, Hamano T. Acute complete bilateral ophthalmoplegia and ptosis without ataxia or areflexia associated with serum anti-GQ 1b antibody. *Neurol. Clin. Neurosci.* 2017. 5(6):178-80. doi: 10.1111/ncn3.12144.

[4] Shumway CL, Motlagh M, Wade M. Anatomy, head and neck, eye extraocular muscles. [Updated 2021 Aug 11]. In: *StatPearls* [Internet]. Treasure Island (FL): StatPearls Publishing; 2021 Jan-.

[5] Haładaj R. Normal Anatomy and Anomalies of the Rectus Extraocular Muscles in Human: A Review of the Recent Data and Findings. *Biomed. Res. Int.* 2019 Dec 28;2019:8909162. doi: 10.1155/2019/8909162.

[6] Arnoldi K. The non-surgical management of ophthalmoplegia. *J. Binocul. Vis. Ocul. Motil.* 2018 Jan-Mar;68(1):24-27. doi: 10.1080/2576117X.2017.1418459.

[7] Chae CS, Kwon KM, Lee JS, Kim YH. A case report of overlapping Miller Fisher syndrome, Guillain-Barré syndrome, and the Bickerstaff brainstem encephalitis. *Neurologist.* 2018 Jul;23(4):128-130. doi: 10.1097/NRL.0000000000000183.

[8] Labodi LD, Adrien M, Anne A, Muhammad K, René D, Bernard B. Miller-fisher syndrome on the borders of guillain-barre syndrome: about one case and review of literature. *Clin. Med. Rep.* 2017;1:1-5.

[9] Kurniawan M, Suharjanti I, Pinzon RT. *Panduan praktik klinis neurologi [Neurological Clinical Practice Guideline].* Jakarta: Perhimpunan Dokter Spesialis Saraf Indonesia. 2016.

[10] Singman EL, Matta NS, Silbert DI. Nonsurgical treatment of neurologic diplopia. *Am. Orthopt. J.* 2013;63:63-8. doi: 10.3368/aoj.63.1.63.

[11] Sehic A, Guo S, Cho KS, Corraya RM, Chen DF, Utheim TP. Electrical Stimulation as a Means for Improving Vision. *Am. J. Pathol.* 2016 Nov;186(11):2783-2797. doi: 10.1016/j.ajpath.2016.07.017.

[12] Rahmatnejad K, Ahmed OM, Waisbourd M, Katz LJ. Non-invasive electrical stimulation for vision restoration: Dream or reality? *Expert Rev. Ophthalmol.* 2016;11(5):325-27.

[13] Arianda R. Physiotherapy management for ptosis with diplopia at RSUP Dr. Sardjito Yogyakarta [dissertation]. Surakarta, Indonesia: Universitas Muhammadiyah Surakarta; 2012.

[14] Liu ZD, Jun Hu, Zhou WK. Electroacupuncture therapy for ophthalmoplegia: a case series. *World J. Acupunct. Moxibustion.* 2017;27(2):6-47.

[15] Putri RA, Santoso TB, Rahman F, OR M, Wijianto SS, Or M. Physiotherapy management for binocular diplopia due to abducens paralysis at RSUP Dr. Sardjito Yogyakarta [dissertation]. Surakarta, Indonesia: Universitas Muhammadiyah Surakarta; 2018.

Chapter 14

Uterine Perforation Caused by Curettage and Undiagnosed Caesarean Scar Pregnancy with Placenta Accreta

Fernandi Moegni[1], M. Syah Reza A[1,*], Noroyono Wibowo[2] and Yuditiya Purwosunu[2]

[1]Department of Obstetrics and Gynecology, Faculty of Medicine, Universitas Indonesia, Jakarta, Indonesia

[2]Fetomaternal Division, Department of Obstetrics and Gynecology, Faculty of Medicine, Universitas Indonesia, Jakarta, Indonesia

Abstract

A caesarean scar pregnancy (CSP) is a severe late complication of caesarean sections (CS) and has a potentially high risk for uterine rupture, intrapartum haemorrhage and maternal mortality. Uterine perforation is a major complication of dilation and curettage (D&C) due to blind uterine manipulation. We present a hypovolemic shock grade IV case due to uterine perforation after curettage of an unknown CSP in a woman who had had two previous CS. The patient, who was three months pregnant, presented with a hypovolemic state due to massive bleeding from a prior curettage procedure. Due to uncontrolled excessive bleeding, we performed a hysterectomy as a life-saving measure. The histological findings showed remnant conception from CSP complicated with placenta accreta spectrum (PAS). Early diagnosis and prompt treatment are crucial to avoid unnecessary complications in the future.

Keywords: caesarean scar pregnancy, uterine rupture, curettage

[*] Corresponding Author's Email: rezaanwar90@gmail.com.

In: The 6th Annual International Conference …
Editors: M. Maidarti, H. Winarto, C. O. M. Jasirwan et al.
ISBN: 978-1-68507-925-3

Introduction

In the last two decades, there has been a significant increase in the number of caesarean sections performed. The caesarean procedure causes subsequent disruption of the endometrial and myometrial lining, which leads to abnormal implantation in the scar. Persistent caesarean scar pregnancy (CSP) increases the risk of uterine rupture, haemorrhage, loss of fertility, maternal mortality and placenta accreta spectrum (PAS). The current literature suggests that persistent CSP and PAS are not two different illnesses but are a result of a single anomaly invading the myometrium early in the first trimester, leading to uterine rupture as the pregnancy progresses [1-4]. There is not enough data to show the possibility of CSP in women with a previous pregnancy, which is frequently mistaken as an aborted pregnancy. Early presentation of PAS in the first-second trimester is less well recognised, as one of the first trimester consequences is CSP. The diagnosis of CSP is challenging, as it can be diagnosed in one of two ways [1-5]:

1. During ultrasound examination in a patient who has had previous caesarean surgery.
2. As a life-threatening situation, as stated in this case report.

Uterine perforation is a significant complication of D&C. Uterine wall defects cause intraabdominal bleeding and trauma. Clinical manifestations such as abdominal discomfort, headache, pulse and reverse abdominal wall pain can occur immediately after D&C or later. Risk factors of uterus perforation include uterus factors (gestation, anatomical variations of the uterus and post-menopausal uterus), surgical management (suction cannula, hegar dilator and curettage) and an inexperienced surgeon [6, 7].

Case Report

Patient Information

A 31-year-old multiparous woman with chief complaint of vaginal bleeding for two hours before being admitted to our emergency room, following a curettage at a previous hospital. The previous hospital diagnosed the patient with an incomplete abortion on G3P2 10 WGA with following two previous CS. Due to indication of vaginal bleeding and abdominal pain, the previous hospital performed a curettage. After the curettage, the patient developed heavier vaginal bleeding and was referred to our hospital.

Clinical Findings

The patient arrived in hypovolemic shock with blood pressure 60/40 mmHg and tachycardia heart rate (123 x/min). We found diffuse abdominal tenderness on physical examination.

Diagnostic Assessment

Laboratory tests revealed a haemoglobin level of 5.9 g/dl. A transabdominal US examination found a hypo and hyperechoic mass between the bladder and anterior uterine wall, which can be seen in Figure 1. The patient was diagnosed with hypovolemic shock grade IV due to vaginal bleeding resulting from suspected uterine perforation following CSP, post curettage at the previous hospital and the previous two CS.

Therapeutic Intervention

We performed resuscitation, prepared 1,000 mL Packed Red Cell and 1,000 mL Fresh Frozen Plasma, and based on a consultation with an anaesthesiologist, an emergency exploration laparotomy was performed.

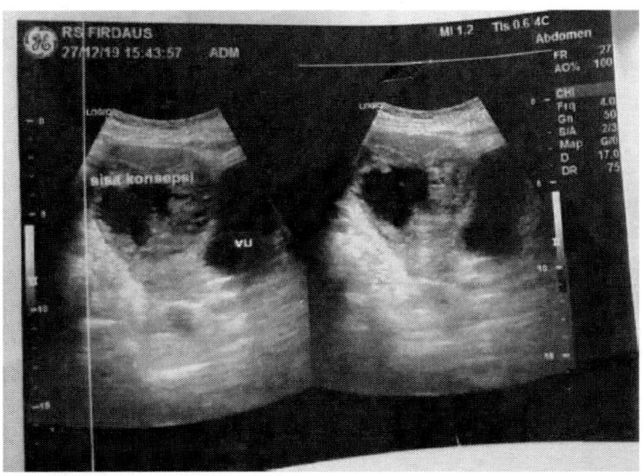

Figure 1. Transabdominal US examination picture.

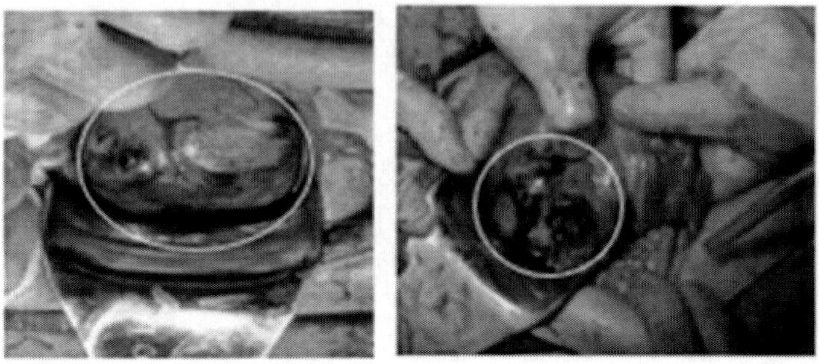

Figure 2. The bluish area extended to the left.

In the intraoperative procedure, we found blood from intraabdominal around 100 ccs, a prominent enlarged 10 x 10 cm fragile bluish area at the whole isthmus part from anterior through posterior, with perforated and active bleeding at the rear part (see Figure 2). We performed a laparotomy with subtotal hysterectomy, and the process was extended into the left parametrial. The estimated total blood loss was 1,500 cc.

Follow-Up and Outcomes

The patient was hospitalised in the ICU for one day and in the ward for the next three days, then discharged. A total of 1,500 mL PRC was given during transfusion. The histological finding was remnant conception from CSP complicated with PAS (see Figure 3).

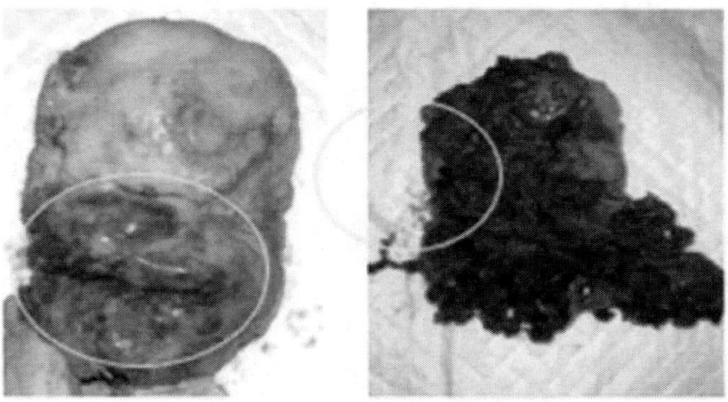

Figure 3. Specimen of uterus (anterior and posterior view).

Discussion

This study was conducted based on the Amendment of the Declaration of Helsinki 2013, and we ensure anonymity of our patient. CSP is the placement of a gestational sac within the scar from prior caesarean surgery. Persistent CSP is a risk for uterine rupture, severe bleeding, infertility and maternal mortality [1-5, 8]. The diagnosis was made based on the patient's history and clinical signs, such as abdominal pain and vaginal bleeding, ranging from spotting to a life-threatening haemorrhage, symptoms and pelvic examination with non-specific findings like vaginal bleeding and abdominal pain. Transvaginal ultrasound was the primary imaging modality with a sensitivity of 84.6%. The diagnosis criteria were as follows:

1. Trophoblast is situated between the bladder and the anterior uterine wall.
2. There are no foetal components in the uterine cavity.
3. The sagittal uterine view showed no myometrium between the gestational sac and urinary bladder (the anterior uterine wall) [4, 9].

A negative *sliding organs sign* (the sliding of any organs such as cervix, the uterine fundus the ovaries, and their possible pathologies relative to the static pelvic wall or the intestines) was found in the ultrasound. Colour doppler imaging and 3-dimensional power Doppler ultrasonography may improve diagnosis accuracy, while evaluating the flow, resistance and pulsatility indices in the peritrophoblastic vasculature. MRI for precise measurement of the distance between the urinary bladder, myometrium and gestational sac offers excellent visibility of the uterine cavity and cervical canal, adjuvant to endovaginal ultrasonography and follow-up [4, 10, 11]. Currently, because of its rarity, there is still no agreement on how to manage CSP. The standard protocol was to terminate the pregnancy as soon as possible after diagnosis. Delaying the procedure will cause complications. Expectant management may result in uterine rupture. Pharmacological treatment could be done by giving methotrexate (MTX). However, systemic MTX can only be used in cases with certain criteria: more than eight weeks of gestation, no sign of foetal cardiac activity and beta-human chorionic gonadotropin (beta-hCG) levels < 12,000 mIU/mL. The aim is to reduce beta-hCG levels by 15% seven days after administration [1, 4, 12].

Furthermore, local MTX has a 61.1% success rate and can be used in pregnancies with beta-HCG < 20,000 mIU/mL and a mass less than 3 cm in diameter of local embryocides. Potassium chloride, crystalline trichosanthin with mifepristone and hyperosmolar glucose have also been used, but with a high failure rate and the need for rescue hysterectomies to control bleeding [4, 12].

The choice of treatments in CSP include D&C, uterine artery embolisation (UAE) coupled with MTX arterial injection, hysteroscopy, resection of CSP through a transvaginal route, laparoscopy and laparotomy. The Triple-P procedure has been proposed as a viable option, particularly in PAS. Under the ultrasound or hysteroscopy direction, local MTX and simultaneous gestational sac aspiration are ideal and minimally invasive [4, 12]. Hysterectomy is performed in emergency conditions (massive bleeding or uterine rupture). D&C has low cost, yet it is suboptimal and has significant risks of bleeding and a low success rate, which means uterine perforation becomes a high risk for hysterectomy and fertility loss. Uterine perforation is a substantial complication of D&C due to blind uterine manipulation. Uterine wall defects cause intraabdominal bleeding and trauma. Clinical manifestations such as abdominal discomfort, headache, palpitation and reverse pain of the abdominal wall can occur immediately after D&C or later. The incidence of uterine perforation with curretage is 16.2%. Most of the perforation site is an anterior wall (40%). And also 13% of the perforation is on the posterior wall. Risk factors for uterine perforation include several uterine factors, such as the age of gestation, anatomical variation of uterus, position and attitude of the uterus, parous uterus and scarred uterus, as well as surgical handling with suction cannula, hegar dilator and curettage. Operator experience is also a risk factor. Management of uterine perforation is based on the instruments used. Hysterectomies are needed in emergency cases such as haemorrhagic shock [4, 6, 12].

Initially, an injury may be detected if the device is extended beyond the uterine limit. Furthermore, resistance to further instrumentation is a strong indicator of uterine perforation. Ultrasonography guidance in skilled hands can lessen the danger of perforation [4, 6, 12].

In this case, the patient was already diagnosed with transabdominal ultrasound, which may lead to misdiagnosis and thus delay treatment. The patient had received curettage at the previous hospital and had blind uterine manipulation, which is a high risk for uterine perforation in patients with CSP. Intraabdominal haemorrhage in this patient was suspected due to uterine perforation; therefore, resuscitation and an emergency laparotomy were performed. On intraoperative findings, a bluish appearance suspected as accreta spectrum was found on the site of uterine perforation.

Conclusion

D&C is a simple management for CSP but had high risk for uterine perforation and lead to shock due to heavy bleeding from the uterus, wedge resection of the gestational sac given better outcome after the operation. Hysterectomy is chosen when the patient had unstable hemodynamic and in emergency condition. CSP can be complicated with morbid placenta adherent as gestational advances because of continuum of the abnormality of implantation and it is given more complication, especially uterine perforation which increased the maternal morbidity and mortality.

Competing Interests

None.

Acknowledgments

This article was presented at the 6th International Conference and Exhibition on Indonesian Medical Education and Research Institute (6th ICE on IMERI), Faculty of Medicine, Universitas Indonesia. We thank the 6th ICE on the IMERI committee, who had supported the peer review and manuscript preparation before submitting it to the journal.

References

[1] Kochevar N., Slutsky E. D., Borella N., Mason R., Hook J. W. V., Patel S. S. The rising triad of cesarean scar pregnancy, placenta percreta and uterine rupture. *Case Rep Obstet Gynecol.* 2018:1-6.

[2] Agha R. A., Borrelli M. R., Farwana R., Koshy K., Fowler A. J., Orgill D. P. The SCARE 2018 statement: updating consensus Surgical CAse REport (SCARE) guidelines. *Int J Surg.* 2018;60:132-36.

[3] Rotas M. A. S. Haberman, Levgur M. Cesarean scar ectopic pregnancies: etiology, diagnosis, and management. *Obstet Gynecol.* 2006;107(6):1373-81.

[4] Mande S., Dank G. A., Shiradkar S., Kaul S. K., Puri C. P. Undiagnosed cesarean scar pregnancy: a nightmare. *J Med Sci.* 2017;4:39-42.

[5] Vial Y., Petignat P., Hohlfeld P. Pregnancy in a cesarean scar. *Ultrasound Obstet Gynecol* 2000;16:592-3.

[6] Timor-Tritsch E., Monteagudo A., Cali G., et al., Cesarean scar pregnancy and early placenta accreta share common histology. *Ultrasound Obstet Gynecol.* 2014;43(4):383-95.

[7] Shakir F., Diab Y. The perforated uterus. *Obstet Gynecol.* 2013;15:256-61.

[8] Tokuda H., Nakago S., Kato H., Oishi T., Kotsuji F. Bleeding in the retroperitoneal space under the broad ligament as a result of uterine perforation after dilatation and curettage: report of a case. *J Obs Gynaecol.* 2017;43(4):779-2.

[9] Zosmer N., Fuller., Shaikh H., Johns J., Ross J. A. Natural history of early first trimester pregnancies implanted in cesarean scars. *Ultrasound Obstet Gynecol.* 2015;46:367-75.

[10] Jurkovic D., Hillaby K., Woelfer B., Lawrence A., Salim R., Elson C. J. First-trimester diagnosis and management of pregnancies implanted into the lower uterine segment cesarean section scar. *Ultrasound Obstet Gynecol.* 2003;21(3):220-7.

[11] Pedraszewski P., Wlazlak E., Surkont G. Caesarean scar pregnancy – a new challenge for obstetricians. *J Ultrason.* 2018;18:56-62.

[12] Lin S. Y., Hsieh C. J., Tu Y. A., Li Y. P., Lee C. N., Hsu W. W., et al., New ultrasound grading system for cesarean scar pregnancy and its implications for management strategies: an observational cohort study. *PLoS One.* 2018;13(8):e0202020

[13] Bodur S., Özdamar Ö., Kılıç S., Gün I. The efficacy of the systemic methotrexate treatment in caesarean scar ectopic pregnancy: a quantitative review of English literature. *J Obstet Gynaecol.* 2015;35(3):290-6.

[14] Zhang Y., Gu Y., Wang J. M., Li Y. Analysis of cases with cesarean scar pregnancy. *J Obstet Gynaecol Res.* 2013;39(1):195e202.

Chapter 15

The Role of Lumbar Sympathetic Block as a Treatment of Complex Regional Pain Syndrome: A Case Report

Andy Andy[1,*] and Pryambodho Pryambodho[1]
[1]Department of Anesthesiology and Intensive Care,
Faculty of Medicine, Universitas Indonesia,
Jakarta, Indonesia

Abstract

A 38-year-old female presented with continuous pain for a year starting in the left toes and sometimes radiating to the left thigh. The pain was described as dull and sometimes accompanied by a burning sensation. We found an oedema on the left cruris and left foot accompanied by redness, tenderness, weakness and temperature asymmetry. The patient was diagnosed with complex regional pain syndrome (CRPS) based on the International Association for the Study of Pain (IASP) and Budapest criteria and underwent a lumbar sympathetic block. During the procedure, injection of the neurolytic and local anaesthetic agent was done with 96% 10 ml alcohol, followed by 0.75% 5 ml ropivacaine into the lateral aspect of vertebral body L3, about ¾ anterior of the vertebral body. The pain was relieved by about 50% and the needle was removed. The patient was evaluated in the general ward for four days with a reduction in the average score on the numeric rating scale (NRS) and was discharged from the hospital with sustained pain relief. This is the first reported case of CRPS treated with a lumbar sympathetic block in Indonesia. Besides its minimal invasiveness, it is a good option for decreasing NRS and increasing quality of life in CRPS patients.

---

* Corresponding Author's Email: andybai78@gmail.com.

In: The 6th Annual International Conference …
Editors: M. Maidarti, H. Winarto, C. O. M. Jasirwan et al.
ISBN: 978-1-68507-925-3

Keywords: lumbar sympathetic block, complex regional pain syndrome, CRPS

Introduction

Complex regional pain syndrome (CRPS) refers to a chronic pain condition that is characterised by progressively worsening spontaneous regional pain without dermatomal distribution [1]. The estimated overall incidence rate was 5.4-26.2 per 100,000 person years [2]. While sympathetic block has a theoretical basis in CRPS, evidence of its benefits mostly comes from case reports and retrospective reviews. We report a case of a patient with CRPS treated with lumbar sympathetic block. This is the first reported case of CRPS treated with lumbar sympathetic block in Indonesia.

Case Report

Patient Information

A 38-year-old female presented with continuous pain for a year starting in the left toes and sometimes radiating to the left thigh. The pain was described as dull and was sometimes accompanied by a burning sensation. The patient had no comorbidities or history of trauma before these symptoms. Eight months before, she was assessed with polyarthritis due to spondyloarthropathy by a rheumatologist and treated with methotrexate for four months, but the symptoms persisted. The patient underwent a non-contrast MRI of the left ankle joint with the results of diffuse cutaneous and subcutaneous oedema of the ankle and distal lower limb, diffuse oedema of the muscle belly of flexor hallucis longus, and no signs of arthritis. She consulted a neurologist who diagnosed her with CRPS and referred her to the medical rehabilitation department to undergo six sessions of physiotherapy, including transcutaneous electrical nerve stimulation (TENS) and laser therapy. Symptoms were relieved for a week and recurred with higher pain intensity. Afterwards, she was referred to our acute pain service (APS) team.

Clinical Findings

The patient was moderately ill. She was alert with a Glasgow Coma Scale of 15, normotensive (112/74mmHg), heart rate 93 beats/minute, normal sinus rhythm, respiratory rate 18/min, afebrile at 36.5°C, numeric rating scale (NRS) 4 and saturating at 97% on room air. Physically, we found an oedema on her left lower limb accompanied by redness, hyperalgesia and allodynia (Figure 1a). The laboratory findings were unremarkable.

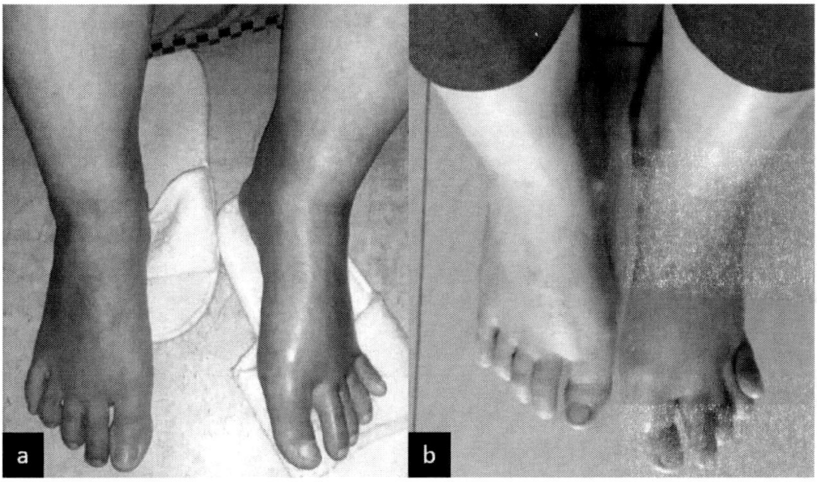

Figure 1. Pictures show the patient with a left lower limb oedema (a), which was reduced after lumbar sympathetic block with alcohol 96% injection (b).

Diagnostic Assessment

Patient was diagnosed with CRPS type 1 based on the International Association for the Study of Pain (IASP) and Budapest criteria for diagnosis of CRPS. All the criteria are based on physical examination without any alteration in laboratory findings. The diagnosis was made after ruling out any joint inflammation, fracture, vascular disorders, peripheral neuropathy or metabolic disorders.

Table 1. Case report timeline

	-8 months	**-4 to -2 months**	**0**	**Hospitalisation**	**+2 to +3 weeks**
Clinical, laboratory and radiological findings	Continuous pain ranging from the left toes, radiating to the left thigh. NRS 4-5 Muscle power 1-2 in the left lower limb	Symptoms were not relieved and were getting worse, NRS 6-7 Left ankle joint MRI: diffuse cutaneous and subcutaneous oedema on distal cruris and ankle, diffuse oedema on FHL muscle belly	Symptoms were relieved for a week, then recurred with higher intensity, NRS 8. Physical examination: oedema on the left lower limb accompanied by redness and hyperalgesia Lab: within normal limit	Pre procedural NRS 6. NRS were reduced >50% after the injection of neurolytic and local anaesthetic agent. NRS 2-3 during evaluation in general ward for 4 days.	NRS during control: 1-2 Reduced swelling Muscle power 3-4 in the left lower limb In week 3, symptoms recurred. NRS 5-6, three episodes of breakthrough pain.

	-8 months	-4 to -2 months	0	Hospitalisation	+2 to +3 weeks
Diagnosis and treatment	Diagnosis: polyarthritis due to spondylo-arthropathy Treatment: Methotrexate 200mg q.i.d	Patient was consulted to a neurologist Diagnosis: CRPS Medication: Aspirin 80mg q.d, methyl-prednisolone 4 mg b.i.d, tramadol 50mg t.i.d, celecoxib 200mg q.d, gabapentin 300mg t.i.d, carbamazepine 200mg t.i.d Patient was consulted to medical rehabilitation department	The patient was consulted to acute pain service Diagnosis: CRPS type 1 The patient was planned to undergo lumbar sympathetic block	Patient was discharged home Medication: Gabapentin 300mg t.i.d, carbamazepine 200mg t.i.d, paracetamol 500mg t.i.d, morphine immediate release 10mg (for break-through pain)	Lumbar sympathetic block Patient was discharged home after pain relief. Medication: Gabapentin 300mg t.i.d, carbamazepine 200mg t.i.d, paracetamol 500mg t.i.d, morphine immediate release 10mg (for break-through pain) Symptom control

Therapeutic Intervention

The patient underwent lumbar sympathetic block after signing the informed consent form. Pre-procedural vital signs were within normal limits and NRS 6. Identification of the lumbar segment was done with fluoroscopy in the prone position.

Puncture with a nerve block needle sized 20G with a needle tip was maintained in the lateral aspect of vertebral body L3, about ¾ anterior of the vertebral body. Confirmed with inferosuperior spread of contrast injection, neurolytic and local anaesthetic agents were administered with 96% 10ml alcohol followed by 0.75% 5ml ropivacaine. The pain was relieved to about half of the prior NRS and the needle was then removed.

Follow-Up and Outcomes

After evaluation in the general ward for four days with an average NRS of 2-3, the patient was discharged. After a week, she went to our outpatient clinic for clinical evaluation and there were improvements such as a reduced pain score, reduced swelling (Figure 1b) and increased muscle power to grade 3-4 in the lower limbs, but she also developed hypoesthesia.

Two weeks later, she was readmitted for the recurrence of symptoms in her left lower limb. We performed the same intervention, which provided sustained relief that lasted four weeks at her last visit to our outpatient clinic.

Patient Perspective

When I was planned for lumbar sympathetic block, I thought I had found a way to reduce the pain I had been feeling. During the injection of those drugs into my nerves, I felt a tremendous pain in my waist like I was being electrocuted, and I screamed. However, after 15-30 minutes, the pain in both my waist and left lower limb gradually disappeared. I am very grateful for the effects of this therapy. Unfortunately, this only lasted two weeks. I have chosen to continue this treatment and will keep looking for treatment options that can relieve this pain for good.

Discussion

This report presents a case of sustained relief after lumbar sympathetic block in a patient with CRPS. In most cases, CRPS occurs when impulses originating from injured body areas strike peripheral nerves and sensitisation centres, where primary afferent nociceptive mechanisms exhibit increased abnormal sensations, including spontaneous pain and hyperalgesia [2].

Lumbar sympathetic blocks can be used to block the nerve supply from the sympathetic chain to the lower extremities. This method is indicated for a group of symptoms associated with the sympathetic nerves, one of which is CRPS. It can be done to reduce pain, accelerate wound healing and avoid amputation [3]. Successful sympathetic block was defined as providing 50% pain relief within six hours. Patients with a 50% reduction in pain for more than six hours are said to have a moderate response. Patients with about 50% reduction in pain for 2-7 days are said to have responded well [4].

The choice of ropivacaine in this case is based on its benefits compared to bupivacaine, such as lower cardiotoxicity and motor block [5]. According to Lew, the characteristics of nerve block caused by ropivacaine are the same or even better than bupivacaine [6]. A meta-analysis conducted by Vinycomb concluded that ropivacaine provides the longest duration of anaesthetic effect on nerve blocks [7]. The use of 96% alcohol in this case is intended for chemical neurolysis, and this agent produces blocks that can last for three to six months. Alcohol is used for protein denaturation, extracting lipid substances, precipitating lipoproteins and mucoproteins, and damaging Schwann cells and neurons, resulting in Wallerian degeneration. Alcohol causes pain on injection, as happened with this patient. Because it is hypobaric and hydrophilic and disperses rapidly from the site of injection, the required volume is also higher at the injection [8]. A literature review by Jain et al. comparing the effects of phenol and alcohol with varying concentrations concluded that 5% phenol has the same neurolytic potential as 40% alcohol. In terms of outcome, phenol causes nerve tissue destruction with a lower intensity and shorter duration of neurolysis than alcohol [9]. In this case, the lumbar sympathetic block relieved the pain for only two weeks. This short duration might be caused by the distribution of neurolytic agents that are more dominant in the psoas muscle compared to the sympathetic chain so that the sympathetic innervation of those undergoing neurolysis is minimal and the nerve regeneration caused nociceptive pain in this patient to recur more quickly. Several factors, such as allodynia, hypoesthesia, and psychological factors, influence the success of sympathetic block; these are negative predictors of chronic CRPS, which does not respond to therapy [10].

Conclusion

Besides its minimal invasiveness, lumbar sympathetic block is an effective treatment for pain control in patients with CRPS. Lumbar sympathetic block is a therapeutic strategy used to avoid amputation, which is associated with a poorer prognosis in CRPS.

Competing Interests

The authors declare that there are no conflicts of interest regarding the publication of this paper.

Acknowledgment

This article was presented at the 6th International Conference and Exhibition on Indonesian Medical Education and Research Institute (6th ICE on IMERI), Faculty of Medicine, Universitas Indonesia. We thank the 6th ICE on the IMERI committee, who had supported the peer review and manuscript preparation for publication to Nova Science Publishers, Inc.

References

[1] Bruehl S. Complex regional pain syndrome. *BMJ.* 2016; 38:82-6.
[2] Petersen PB, Mikkelsen KL, Lauritzen JB, Krogsgaard MR. Risk factors for post-treatment complex regional pain syndrome (CRPS): An analysis of 647 cases of CRPS from the Danish Patient Compensation Association. *Pain Pract.* 2018; 18:341-9.
[3] An JW, Koh JC, Sun JM, Park JY, Choi JB, Shin MJ, Lee YW. Clinical identification of the vertebral level at which the lumbar sympathetic ganglia aggregate. *Korean J Pain.* 2016; 29(2):103-9.
[4] van Eijs F, Geurts J, van Kleef M, Faber CG, Perez RS, Kessels AGH, van Zundert J. Predictors of pain-relieving response to sympathetic blockade in complex regional sain syndrome type 1. *Anesthesiol.* 2012; 116(1):113-21.

[5] Kaur A, Singh RB, Tripathi RK, Choubey S. Comparison between bupivacaine and ropivacaine in patients undergoing forearm surgeries under axillary brachial plexus block: A prospective randomized study. *J Clin Diagn Res*. 2015; 9(1):101-6.

[6] Lew E, Vloka JD, Hadzic A. Ropivacaine for peripheral nerve blocks: Are there advantages? *Pain Manag*. 2001; 5(2):56-9.

[7] Vinycomb TI, Sahhar LJ. Comparison of local anesthetics for digital nerve blocks: A systematic review. *J Hand Surg*. 2014; 39(4):744-51.

[8] Koyyalagunta D, Engle MP, Yu J, Feng L, Novy DM. The effectiveness of alcohol versus phenol based splanchnic nerve neurolysis for the treatment of intra-abdominal cancer pain. *Pain Phys*. 2016; 19:281-92.

[9] Jain S, Gupta R. Neural blockade with neurolytic agents. *Pain Manag*. 2007; (32):343-8.

[10] Hartrick CT, Kovan JP, Naismith P. Outcome prediction following sympathetic block for complex regional pain syndrome. *Pain Pract*. 2004; 4(3):222-8.

Chapter 16

The Socratic Method on How to Deal with Guilt in Severe Depressive Episodes with Psychotic Symptoms and Other Habits and Impulse Disorder Due to Excessive Masturbation: A Case Report

Emilya Kusnaidi[1,*] and Heriani Tobing[1]

[1]Department of Psychiatry, Faculty of Medicine Universitas Indonesia
Cipto Mangunkusumo General Hospital,
Jakarta, Indonesia

Abstract

Excessive guilt can lead to depressive tendencies if it is not addressed. While most guilt is internal, it is conditioned by external stimuli, which implies it may be unlearned with the appropriate behaviours. Detecting this connection is the first step in breaking the cycle. Depression is anticipated to overtake anxiety as the most frequent mental condition, and cognitive behavioural therapy (CBT) is suggested as an effective treatment for depression. Through Socratic questioning, patients learn to identify and justify their intuitions and assumptions. Socratic enquiry requires patients to account for themselves: their ideas, behaviours and beliefs.

The therapist's role is to dispute the logic of numerous and multifarious ideas and cognitive errors. Thus, the goal of Socratic enquiry is to uncover the reasons and assumptions that patients rely on to live their lives.

---

* Corresponding Author's Email: mei.kusnaidi@gmail.com.

In: The 6th Annual International Conference …
Editors: M. Maidarti, H. Winarto, C. O. M. Jasirwan et al.
ISBN: 978-1-68507-925-3

Our patient had a severe depressive episode with psychotic symptoms and other habit and impulse disorders due to excessive masturbation for the last seven months. The patient was treated with behavioural therapy at first. After 12 CBT with Socratic questioning sessions, the patient became conscious of automatic thoughts and learned to replace them with alternative thoughts. He also improved his ability to perceive and communicate his feelings. The severity of his depression symptoms decreased, and he was able to enhance his involvement in everyday activities.

Keywords: Socratic questioning, cognitive behavioural therapy, depression, guilt

Introduction

The Socratic Method is named after Socrates, a Greek Athenian philosopher who avoided using direct teaching in favour of using enquiry to inspire students to come to their own conclusions and question prevailing opinions. Nowadays, the method is characterised as a form of discovery in which the therapist asks a series of methodically sequenced questions to help clarify issues and identify thoughts, assumptions and beliefs. The therapist also evaluates the meaning of events and assesses certain thoughts or behaviours related to it [1].

The Socratic technique is widely used in the field of psychotherapy. It has been used to treat depression, psychosis and personality disorders, as well as specific issues [2].

Our patient had a severe depressive episode with psychotic symptoms and other habit and impulse disorders due to excessive masturbation for the last seven months. While most guilt is internal, excessive guilt can lead to depressive tendencies if it is not addressed.

Although Socratic questioning is extensively addressed in the psychotherapy literature, there does not appear to be a widely agreed definition of the approach, and there are discrepancies, mistakes and inconsistencies surrounding its use.

Case Report

Patient Information

A 30-year-old unmarried Moslem male came to the outpatient clinic. He came into therapy with complaints of being restless, feeling guilty and sinful due to excessive masturbation. He also complained about not being able to socialise with his family and colleagues.

He was raised in a family with strong religious views, and conversations about sex were taboo in the family. It began in 2012, when the patient started experimenting with his sexuality.

The idea of masturbation came from his circle of friends. He recognised that masturbation could make him feel good. Since then, whenever he felt sad, lonely, or bored, he watched porn videos and masturbated to feel better about himself. The patient did this every day.

Clinical Findings

Current symptom presentation: dysphoric mood with constricted affect, history of commanding type auditoric hallucination, preoccupation about masturbating while watching porn, and he had the automatic thoughts and cognitive errors shown in Table 1.

Table 1. The Patient's Automatic Thoughts and Cognitive Errors

Automatic thoughts	Cognitive errors
'Sex is sin' 'Masturbation is sin' 'Watching porn video is sin' 'Sex before marriage is sin' 'I'm a sinner'	• Fortune telling: 'I managed to stop watching porn videos before, so now I can definitely stop whenever I want it.' 'When I try to make conversations with my family, they will ignore me.' 'My friends won't relate to my stories if I talk about one.' • Labelling 'I'm an introvert' 'I'm awkward at socialising' 'I can't open a conversation'

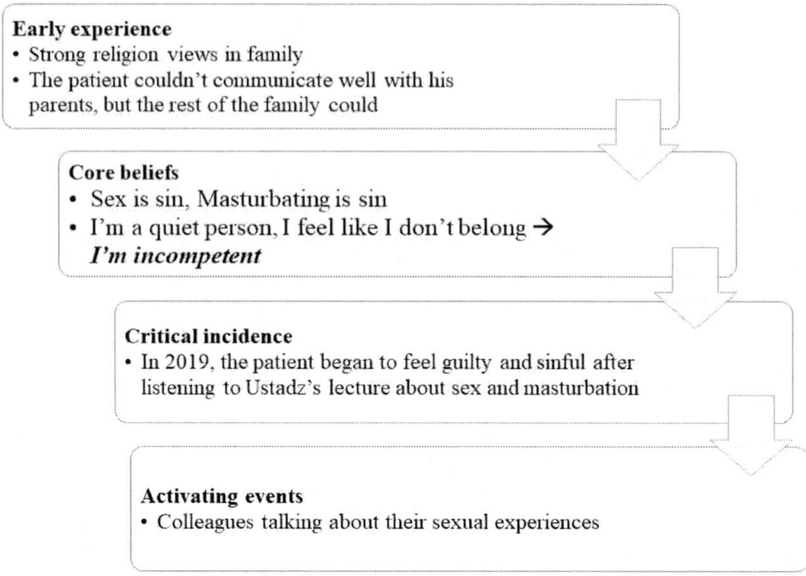

Figure 1. Functional analysis of the patient.

Timeline

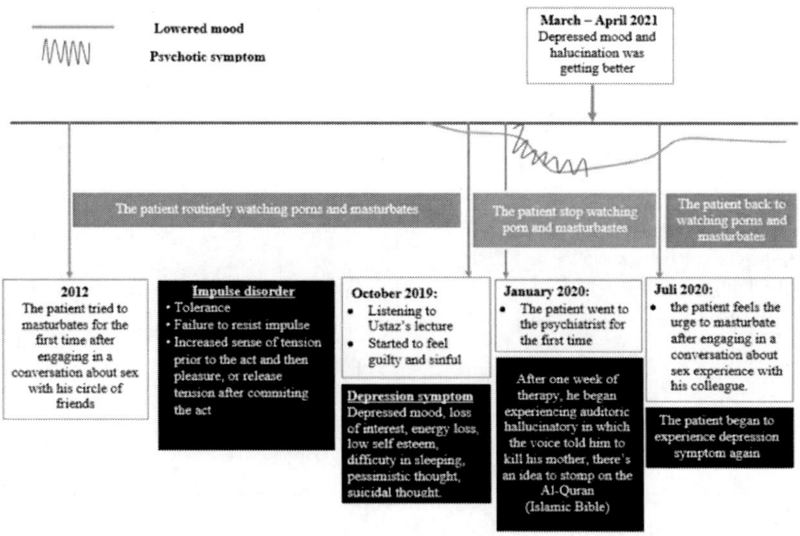

Figure 2. Timeline and course of illness.

Diagnostic Assessment

The author carried out the assessment at the outpatient clinic via an unstructured interview with the patient. The interview was conducted to explore the patient's background as well as his psychiatric and sexual history. At first, the patient was reluctant to describe his sexual history due to his Eastern cultural background, in which it is somewhat taboo to talk about sexual experiences.

However, after developing a good therapeutic alliance, the patient was willing to talk about it. We applied the ICD-10 criteria to the patient's condition.

He was then diagnosed with severe depressive episodes with psychotic symptoms and other habit and impulse disorders. Imaging and laboratory testing were not applied in this case as they were not necessary for the patient's condition.

Therapeutic Intervention

The patient was treated with Fluoxetine 1 x 50 mg, Aripiprazole 1 x 5 mg and Cognitive Behavioural Therapy (CBT) through Socratic questioning. With this method, at first the patient struggled to identify and defend their intuitions, beliefs and assumptions.

The therapist challenged him with facts and disputation of his thoughts and beliefs. Socratic enquiry aims to reveal the ideas and assumptions upon which the patients lead their lives and come to alternative ones. Thus, hopefully it will also change their behaviour.

Follow-Up and Outcomes

After 12 sessions of CBT with Socratic questioning, the patient became aware of automatic thoughts and learned to find alternative thoughts. Once he earned the skills of finding alternative thoughts, the suffering from guilty feelings was slowly reduced.

He also learned to recognise and express his emotions in a better way. He started socialising with his family and friends. The severity of his depression symptoms decreased, and he was able to enhance his involvement in everyday activities.

Patient's Perspective

The patient felt that the therapy worked. He continued to use the strategies he learned during therapy and found that his behaviour was controllable. He also had a good relationship with his family.

Discussion

When working with patients from diverse cultural backgrounds, a Socratic approach may be less useful because it is more likely to be regarded as a judgement of their thoughts, feelings and behaviours. CBT is beneficial for a wide spectrum of mental problems. However, when the therapist is non-judgmental and willing to know the patient's background, it can appear that the patient feels that he was understood, thus making a good therapeutic alliance. With this form of alliance, the therapist can challenge the patient's thoughts, feelings and perceptions so the patient realises their automatic thoughts and learns to replace them with alternative ones.

Conclusion

Socratic questioning is effective in reducing patients' suffering from guilty feelings and increasing the capacity to find an alternative thought. A good therapeutic alliance and a non-judgmental and open-minded therapist are important factors to make the patient comfortable to follow the therapeutic session.

Competing Interests

No potential competing interest was reported by the authors.

Acknowledgment

This article was presented in the 6th International Conference and Exhibition on Indonesian Medical Education and Research Institute (6th ICE on IMERI),

Faculty of Medicine, Universitas Indonesia. We thank the 6th ICE on IMERI committee, who had supported the peer-review and manuscript preparation for publication to Nova Science Publishers, Inc.

References

[1] Clark GI, Egan SJ. The Socratic method in cognitive behavioural therapy: A narrative review. *Cognit Ther Res.* 2015; 39(6):863-79.

[2] Beck S. *Cognitive behaviour therapy: Basics and beyond.* 2nd ed. New York: The Gillford Press; 2011.

Chapter 17

Clinical Outcome of Nutritional Support in an Elderly Patient with Laryngeal Cancer After Chemoradiation Therapy: A Case Report

Thia Juniaty Manik*, **Diyah Eka Andayani and Nurul Ratna Mutu Manikam**
Department of Nutrition, Faculty of Medicine, University of Indonesia,
Dr Cipto Mangunkusumo Hospital, Jakarta, Indonesia

Abstract

The increase in life expectancy has led to a higher number of elderly patients with head and neck cancer (HNC). Weight loss is more common in HNC patients even after therapy. Eating problems may persist after treatment is completed. The elderly may be more susceptible to chemoradiation toxicity because of the reduction of physiological function. The patient was a 60-year-old man with laryngeal squamous cell carcinoma (SCC), cancer cachexia, post 5 cycles of chemotherapy and intensity modulated-radiation therapy in 35 fractions. He had lost 8.1 kg (17%) during chemoradiation, refused nasogastric tube insertion and developed severe malnutrition. There was a decrease in the estimated glomerular filtration rate (eFGR) after chemotherapy. The patient had eating difficulty because of dysgeusia and missing teeth. He had home visits including assessment of nutritional complaints due to therapy, anthropometrics, body composition, intake analysis, handgrip strength, functional capacity and nutritional prescriptions. His intake increased gradually, his body weight increased by 5 kg after three monitoring sessions, and his renal function improved slightly. Among older adults

* Corresponding Author's Email: tjmanik@gmail.com.

In: The 6th Annual International Conference …
Editors: M. Maidarti, H. Winarto, C. O. M. Jasirwan et al.
ISBN: 978-1-68507-925-3

with HNC, it is important to improve nutritional status through nutritional therapy after chemoradiation. However, doing so is quite challenging due to the side effects that may linger beyond the treatment period.

Keywords: head and neck cancer, nutritional support, cachexia

Introduction

More than half of new squamous cell carcinomas (SCCs) in head and neck cases are diagnosed in older people, and the prevalence is expected to rise by more than 10% in 15 years [1]. The elderly may be more susceptible to chemoradiation toxicity because of reduction of physiological function. In the majority of patients, eating problems persisted after treatment was completed.2 Pain and difficulty in chewing and swallowing were noted after one month in 70% of patients and after six months in 65% of patients. These symptoms also had a significant effect on oral intake [2, 3]. One of the goals of post-treatment follow-up is the evaluation of treatment-related complications.

Most head and neck cancer (HNC) patients who have undergone radiotherapy suffer from altered taste and reduced food intake. The return of taste was observed as soon as four to five weeks post radiotherapy completion [4]. Chemotherapy agents may improve cancer control, but they have various sides effects [5]. Various renal toxicity was attributed to multiple chemotherapy agents.

Caring for people with cancer does not end when active treatment does. Patients are often left with many physical sequalae, most of which gradually resolve. During this time, abundant support is needed – which in some cases is lacking [6].

Nutrition is an important aspect in multimodal cancer care; however, nutrition support is not routinely provided in cancer patients after treatment. We describe a case of HNC in an elderly patient after chemoradiation, providing insights into treatments with nutritional therapy. It is expected that nutrition therapy may improve nutritional status after chemoradiation.

Case Report

Patient Information

A 60-year-old male patient with laryngeal SCC post tracheostomy and total laryngectomy was first consulted at the Clinical Nutrition Clinic in the Radiotherapy Department due to weight loss of 14.6 kg (24%) in more than one year, with a malnutrition screening tool (MST) score of 3 (considered malnutrition). The patient was planned to undergo chemoradiation. He had risk factors for cancer, including age, male gender and previous smoking habit. He was married and had two children, and he had been unemployed since his illness. He had no previous history of other diseases. Pre-radiation monitoring after consultation with a clinical nutrition physician showed an increase in body weight (BW) from 45.5 to 46.3 kg.

Seven of the patient's teeth were extracted prior to the initiation of radiotherapy. The patient had worn dentures for the upper teeth before this illness. The patient underwent five cycles of chemotherapy and intensity-modulated radiation therapy in 35 fractions. Monitoring was carried out once a week while undergoing chemoradiation. He experienced side effects, including pain when swallowing, dry mouth and reduced taste. He refused to have a nasogastric tube. His BW decreased by 5.2 to 41.1 kg at the seventh week of monitoring and to 38.2 kg two weeks after chemoradiation. There had been a decrease in eFGR since the fifth week of monitoring. After completing chemoradiation, the patient could not see the clinical nutrition physician regularly because the health insurance did not cover the treatment. Considering his nutritional status and eating difficulty, the patient decided to have a home care visit.

Clinical Findings

At the first home visit, he had experienced difficulty defecating for four days. His stomach felt bloated and his food intake had decreased. It took a long time for him to chew foods because of his missing teeth. He felt less pain in swallowing, but food remained flavourless. The skin on the neck looked blackish and he showed signs of severe malnutrition, such as loss of subcutaneous fat overlying the ribs and wasting in the extremities. His height was 165 cm, and his BW increased 0.2 kg to 38.4 kg within three weeks, compared to the last follow-up at the outpatient visit. Body composition measurement used BIA Omron® HBF 375 showed a slight increase in muscle mass (Table 1).

Table 1. Changes in the patient's clinical findings

Variable	**Outpatient Service (last visit)**	**Home Care Visit**		
		1	**2**	**3**
Complaints	Decreased appetite, tasteless	Less pain when swallowing, tasteless, need more time for chewing. Blackish skin on radiation site	Need more time for chewing. Neck stiffness	Need more time for chewing. Neck stiffness, lump on neck
Functional Capacity	ECOG score 1	ECOG score 1	ECOG score 1	ECOG score 1
Hand Grip (kg) Right Left	 36.2 38	 33.6 40.9	 35.3 39.1	 36.7 40.1
Anthropometry: BW (kg) BMI (kg/m^2)	 38.2 14	 38.4 14.1	 42.2 15.5	 43.4 15.9
Body Composition: Muscle mass (32.9-38.9%) Fat mass (10 – < 20%) FFMI (ε17 kg/m^2)	 30 (⊔) 13.8 (normal) 11.7(↓)	 31.9(⊔) 13.5 (normal) 12.2(⊔)	 33.2 (normal) 11.2 (normal) 13.8(⌟)	 30.8(⊔) 18.0 (normal) 13.1(⊔)

BW: Body Weight; FFMI: Fat Free Mass Index; BMI: Body Mass Index.

The patient's intake in his first visit to the outpatient clinic before a home care visit was 1,932 kcal, which decreased during chemotherapy to a range of 1,164-1,760 kcal (Table 2), 28-40 kcal/kg/d and protein 0.4-1.3 gram/kg.d. The intake in week seven of chemoradiation was 1,164 kcal, which was the patient's lowest intake. The main intake was from a liquid diet, such as home-made liquid food and oral nutrition supplement (ONS).

The energy intake in the first home care visit was (Table 2) 1,403 kcal (37 kcal/kg/d) and protein 51 g (1.3 g/kg/d). The patient consumed liquid and soft food from baby cereals and biscuits, olive oil, milk and ONS. He could not meet the prescription given previously due to painful swallowing and altered taste.

Table 2. Energy intake and prescription

Variable	Chemo Radiation Intake	Home Care					
		I1	P1	I2	P2	I3	P3
Energy (kcal)	1,164-1,760	1,403	1,636	2,055	2,048	2,220	2,176
Energy (kcal/kg BW)	28-40	37	43	49	49	51	50
Protein (g)	18-65	51	49	44	51	55	57
Protein (g/kgBW)	0.4-1.3	1.3	1.3	1	1.2	1.3	1.3
Fat (%)	21-32	31	34	32	36	35	34
Carbohydrate (%)	53-70	54	54	59	54	55	56

I: Patient Intake; P: Prescriptions.

Timeline

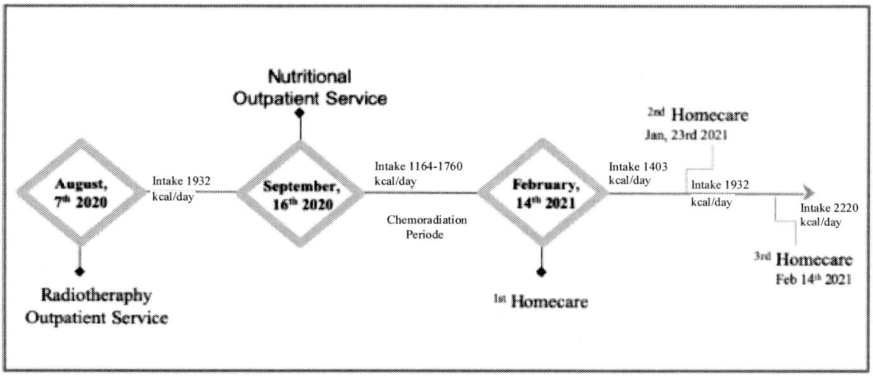

Figure 1. Timeline of the study.

Diagnostic Assessment

The patient was diagnosed with severe malnutrition based on ASPEN criteria. He met three of six criteria, had a 25% weight loss in the last year, food intake less than 75% of the estimated energy requirement, and decreased muscle and fat mass. Cachexia diagnosis was met from fatigue, anorexia and low FFMI. Laboratory results showed a suspected acute kidney injury (AKI).

Therapeutic Intervention

At each home care visit, we provided personalised dietary guidance and dietary prescriptions (Table 2). The energy need for this patient was measured by the Harris-Benedict formula with a stress factor of 2. In the first home care, the total energy requirement was 2,012 kcal. Nutritional therapy was initiated with a diet of 1,636 kcal/day and protein intake of 1.3 gram/kg/d. Protein were adjusted according to kidney function. Nutritional intake was given with more than 50% liquid food. Diet was prescribed and adjusted to patient preference with porridge or baby cereal, packaged cereal, biscuit, egg, fruit juice, milk (3x120 kcal), oral nutritional support (2x190 kcal) and olive oil (3x50 kcal). He still consumed a lot of simple carbohydrates. He preferred baby cereals or packaged cereal to rice porridge or other homemade foods because he felt tired of prolonged chewing.

The patient was encouraged to consume a variety of fruits and a food source of branch chain amino acid (BCAA) from protein and omega-3 fatty acid in liquid preparation to increase the patient's adherence. In addition to normal daily activities, 30 minutes of exercise was also recommended.

Follow-Up and Outcomes

During follow-up, the patient's intake increased gradually. Protein intake had not reached the target in the second visit. The patient could taste food better. BW increased by 5 kg after three monitoring sessions. Body composition showed that the patient's FFMI, muscle mass and body fat percentage increased to 13.1 kg/m2, 13.4 kg and 18%, respectively, compared to the last monitoring at the outpatient clinic. The patient was advised to reduce cereal and biscuits and to start adding other foods from original sources, such as boiled potatoes, fish or tofu. The foods could be processed into soft meals to help with the difficulty of chewing. In the second visit, eGFR was checked and it showed slight improvement (Table 3).

Table 3. Laboratory results

Laboratory	**W-1**	**W-2**	**W-3**	**W-4**	**W-5**	**W-6**	**W-7**	**W-10**	**HC**
eGFR	72.6	-	81.4	54.2	50	46.1	40	50	58
Creatinine	1.1	-	1	1.4	1.5	1.6	1.8	1.49	1.32

Note: W = week.

Patient Perspective

Home care visits had a positive effect on the patient. The patient was happy and motivated to reverse his weight loss. Nutritional intervention helped him optimise his nutritional status.

Discussion

This case report introduced an elderly patient who underwent nutritional therapy at home due to severe malnutrition after chemoradiation. The patient had difficulties eating because of dysgeusia and missing teeth. During therapy, the patient developed AKI. The patient's intake increased gradually; BW increased by 5 kg during home care visits and renal function improved. The patient's FFMI, muscle mass and body fat percentage had increased compared to the last monitoring at the outpatient visit.

In cachectic patients, varying degrees of weight loss occur together with metabolic abnormalities, loss of skeletal muscle and lipolysis. Approximately 50% of all cancer patients who had decreasing body mass were found to be more hypermetabolic compared to the control, providing they have similar body composition, physical activity, weight loss and age [7, 8]. Unhealthy teeth extraction prior to radiotherapy and unawareness of nutritional problems may provide iatrogenic causes of weight loss [9].

Zietarska et al., [10] showed nutritional status improvement in the high protein ONS group (one drink contains 18 g protein) compared to the control group. No changes were observed in performance status or quality of life during nutritional support. Waitzberg et al., [11] highlighted the importance of emphasising the use of ONS in the home care environment.

ESPEN recommended increased oral intake as a nutritional intervention in malnourished cancer patients. This includes offering ONS and encouraging the intake of protein- and energy-dense food and fluid that is well tolerated. The recommended amount of energy intake for cancer patients is generally between 25 kcal and 30 kcal/(kg/d) with adjustment for underweight. Daily protein intake must be above 1 g/kg and up to 1.5 g/kg when possible [12]. Patients with acute or chronic kidney failure protein supply should not exceed a daily intake of more than 1.0 or 1.2 g/kg, respectively [13].

In the second and third visits, the patient's appetite was better, but he preferred simple carbohydrates and packaged foods to healthy carbohydrates. During all phases of cancer survival, the principles outlined in the American

Cancer Society Guidelines on Nutrition and Physical Activity for Cancer Prevention should be regarded as the basis for a healthy diet [14]. Long term health depends heavily on type of fat, protein or carbohydrate. Healthy carbohydrate choices are those that come from foods rich in nutrients essential to health, such as phytochemicals, and fibres that normally can be obtained from whole grains, legumes, vegetables and fruit. Nutrient-poor, low fibre and carbohydrate-rich foods simply add calories to the diet and should only make up a small amount of the diet.

Not all chemotherapy patients eventually had kidney injury. In this patient, as a result of age-related changes in pharmacokinetics and pharmacodynamics, carboplatin use may have an effect on his kidneys. The omission of some chemotherapeutics or reduced renal blood flow may be the cause of physiological decline in glomerular filtration rate.1 Serum creatinine level is not a sensitive indicator of renal function in the elderly.

Chemotherapy toxicity and mortality amongst cancer patients can be independently predicted by progressive loss of skeletal muscle. Diminishment of FFM may be accompanied by fat mass loss and can be masked by unchanged body weight. During recovery, weight increase can be pointed out by an increase in mass of fat rather than fat-free mass, as seen in the body composition of this patient in third home care visit [15].

Another important component is protein quality. Nutritional strategies to minimise muscle protein loss in adults have also emphasised the usage of high-quality protein with a higher content of indispensable amino acids. Distribution pattern of proteins on meals can increase muscle synthesis and lean mass synthesis in older adults [16]. Body composition evaluation may help document how efficient nutritional support is during a patient's follow up following numerous clinical problems [17]. This patient needs ongoing monitoring including body composition examination to improve his weight and reduce his muscle mass loss that is not limited to three home visits, which becomes the limitation in our case.

To stimulate muscle mass synthesis, physical function and metabolic patterns, ESPEN recommended increased or maintained levels of physical activity. Personalised resistance exercise is suggested in concordance with aerobic exercise [12]. Exercise should also be encouraged for this patient because he has nothing else on which to spend his time.

Conclusion

Follow-up of HNC patients is necessary to monitor treatment effects, nutritional status maintenance and provision of adequate clinical care to minimise side effects, including nutritional intervention. A multidisciplinary care approach including nutrition may be more relevant.

Competing Interests

There is no conflict of interest in publishing this article.

Acknowledgments

This article was presented at the 6th International Conference and Exhibition on Indonesia Medical Education and Research Institute (6th ICE on IMERI), Faculty of Medicine, Universitas Indonesia. We thank the 6th ICE on the IMERI committee, who had supported the peer review and manuscript preparation before submitting it to the journal.

References

[1] Szturz, P., and J. B. Vermorken. 2016. "Treatment of Elderly Patients with Squamous Cell Carcinoma of the Head and Neck." *Frontiers in Oncology* 6:199.

[2] Larsson, M., B. Hedelin, I. Johansson, and E. Athlin. 2005. "Eating Problems and Weight Loss for Patients With Head and Neck Cancer: A Chart Review From Diagnosis Until One Year After Treatment." *Cancer Nursing* 28(6):425–35.

[3] Gorenc, M., N. R. Kozjek, and P. Strojan. 2015. "Malnutrition and Cachexia in Patients with Head and Neck Cancer Treated with (Chemo)Radiotherapy." *Reports of Practical Oncology & Radiotherapy* 20(4):249–58.

[4] Deshpande, T. S., P. Blanchard, L. Wang, R. L. Foote, X. Zhang, and S. J. Frank. 2018. "Radiation-Related Alterations of Taste Function in Patients With Head and Neck Cancer: A Systematic Review." *Current Treatment Options in Oncology* 19(12):72.

[5] Dehkordi, A. H., B. Keikhaei, M. Bahadoram, S. Razmjoo, and M. Barahman. 2020. "Keep the Corners; Impact of Chemotherapy on Renal Function." *Journal of Nephropathology* 9(1):e01

[6] Ganz, P. A. 2009. "Quality of Care and Cancer Survivorship: The Challenge of Implementing the Institute of Medicine Recommendations." *Jounal of Oncology Practice* 5(3):101–5.

[7] Toomey, D., H. P. Redmond, and Bouchier-Hayes D. 1995. "Mechanisms Mediating Cancer Cachexia." *Cancer* 76(12):2418–26.

[8] Lucia, S., M. Esposito, F. R. Fanelli, and M. Muscaritoli. 2012. "Cancer Cachexia: From Molecular Mechanisms to Patient's Care." *Critical Reviews on Oncologenesis* 17(3):315–21.

[9] Lee, H., C. Havrila, V. Bravo, K. Shantz, K. Diaz, J. Larner, et al. 2008. "Effect of Oral Nutritional Supplementation on Weight Loss and Percutaneous Endoscopic Gastrostomy Tube Rates in Patients Treated with Radiotherapy for Oropharyngeal Carcinoma." *Support Care Cancer* 16(3):285–9.

[10] Ziętarska, M., J. Krawczyk-Lipiec, L. Kraj, R. Zaucha, S. Małgorzewicz. 2017. "Chemotherapy-Related Toxicity, Nutritional Status and Quality of Life in Precachectic Oncologic Patients With, or Without, High Protein Nutritional Support. A Prospective, Randomized Study." *Nutrients* 9(10):1108.

[11] Waitzberg, D. L., J. E. De Aguilar-Nascimento, M. C. Gonçalves Dias, N. Pinho, R. Moura, and M. I. T. D. Correia. 2017. "Hospital and Homecare Malnutrition and Nutritional Therapy, in Brazil. Strategies for Alleviating it: A Position Paper." *Nutricion Hospitalaria* 34(4).

[12] Muscaritoli, M., J. Arends, P. Bachmann, V. Baracos, N. Barthelemy, H. Bertz, et al. 2021."ESPEN Practical Guideline: Clinical Nutrition in Cancer." *Clinical Nutrition* 40(5):2898–913.

[13] Arends J, P. Bachmann, V. Baracos, N. Barthelemy, H. Bertz H, F. Bozzetti, et al. 2017. "ESPEN Guidelines on Nutrition in Cancer Patients." *Clinical Nutrition* 36(1):11–48.

[14] Brown J. K., T. Byers, C. Doyle, K. S. Courneya, W. Demark-Wahnefried, L. H. Kushi, et al. 2003. "Nutrition and Physical Activity During and After Cancer Treatment: An American Cancer Society Guide for Informed Choices." *A Cancer Journal for Clinician* 53(5):268–91.

[15] Ræder H., C. Henriksen, S. K. Bøhn, A-ROF Vilbo, H. B. Henriksen, A. S. Kværner, et al. 2018. "Agreement between PG-SGA Category and Fat-Free Mass in Colorectal Cancer Patients." *Clinical Nutrition ESPEN* 27:24–31.

[16] Tomé, D. 2017. "Muscle Protein Synthesis and Muscle Mass in Healthy Older Men." *The Journal of Nutrition* 147(12):2209–11.

[17] Thibault, R., and C. Pichard. 2012. "The Evaluation of Body Composition: A Useful Tool for Clinical Practice." *Annal of Nutrition and Metabolic* 60(1):6–16.

Chapter 18

Effectiveness of Dexamethasone as an Adjuvant in QL Block for Prolonging Analgesia Post-Caesarean Section up to 72 Hours: A Case Series

Natalia Frederika Darmawan Adji Saroso[1]
and Irma Lusiana Tantri[2,*]
[1]Faculty of Medicine, Pelita Harapan University, Tangerang, Indonesia
[2]Anesthesiology Department, Siloam Hospitals Lippo Village, Tangerang, Indonesia

Abstract

Background: Post-caesarean pain is usually associated with persistent pain, increased opioid use, delayed functional recovery and increased risk of postpartum depression. The quadratus lumborum (QL) block is a regional truncal nerve block that has been known for its effectiveness for post-caesarean pain control for up to 48 hours. This study investigates whether the use of dexamethasone as an adjuvant in QL block is effective in providing pain relief for up to 72 hours. *Case Presentation:* This study included four gravida patients who underwent caesarean sections and were anaesthetised through spinal anaesthesia. After the surgery, ultrasound-guided posterior QL block was performed with isobaric Bupivacaine 0.25% 20 ml, lidocaine 2% 5 ml, epinephrine 1:200,000 and dexamethasone 5 mg given on each side. All patients received multimodal analgesia for the first 48 h post-operatively with acetaminophen IV 1,000 mg every eight hours, and ketoprofen suppository 100 mg every 12 hours. The numeric rating scale (NRS) for pain every six hours (for the first 72 hours) and opioid consumption

* Corresponding Author's Email: irmalusianatantri@gmail.com.

In: The 6th Annual International Conference …
Editors: M. Maidarti, H. Winarto, C. O. M. Jasirwan et al.
ISBN: 978-1-68507-925-3

during the first 48 hours was also recorded. *Management and Outcome:* All patients received sufficient pain control for up to 72 hours, with no additional opioid consumption during the first 48 hours. No adverse or unanticipated events occurred. *Conclusion:* A posterior QL block with the addition of dexamethasone as an adjuvant was effective in providing pain relief for up to 72 h post-caesarean section.

Keywords: dexamethasone, postoperative analgesia, quadratus lumborum block, caesarean section, case series

Introduction

Effective postoperative analgesia is essential in patients who have undergone a caesarean section. Besides the safety of the mother and the child, the primary concern of the patients was the pain experienced during or after the surgery. In a caesarean section, there are two components of pain: somatic and visceral. Somatic pain originates from the incision site (Pfannenstiel), which is innervated by the L1 dermatome. Visceral pain originates from cutting the abdominal wall and uterine structures innervated by the hypogastric inferior plexus entering the spinal cord on the T10-L1 nerve fibres [1]. Undertreated pain is associated with persistent discomfort, higher dose opioid requirement, delayed functional recovery and the incidence of postpartum depression. Adequate post-caesarean pain control supports early mobilisation and supports mother-infant interaction to help initiate early breastfeeding [2, 3].

The quadratus lumborum (QL) block was first introduced in 2007 to provide adequate visceral analgesia as a variation of the transversus abdominis plane (TAP) block [4, 5]. The local anaesthetic (LA) spreads to the posterior side of the QL muscle and extends to the middle layer of the thoracolumbar fascia [6, 7]. While the TAP block only has somatic pain coverage, the QL block covers both somatic and visceral pain. The discrepancy might be explained by the spread of LA to the thoracolumbar fascia, as LA blocks impulses from the dense sympathetic nerve fibres that penetrate this structure [8]. Blanco discovered a significant reduction in morphine consumption and lower visual analogue scores (VAS) 48 hours following QL block administration compared to a TAP block [6, 7]. Therefore, QL block is recommended as part of multimodal analgesia in the post-caesarean section [6].

Earlier studies have shown that the addition of corticosteroids to various LA blocks produced a prolonged regional block duration [9, 10]. However, prior studies of dexamethasone as an adjuvant in regional block had a postoperative evaluation period of only up to 48 h. The prolongation of analgesia for up to 72 h due to additional of 10 mg dexamethasone (5 mg on each side) after caesarean section still needs to be determined. This study determines the effectiveness of dexamethasone as an adjuvant in QL block for prolonging post-caesarean pain relief for up to 72 h.

Case Series

This study included four gravida patients of 28-, 31-, 34-, and 23-year-old females who presented for caesarean sections. The patients reported that they had no previous history of hospitalisation or surgery except for the first patient who underwent an emergency caesarean section due to secondary arrest of dilatation. They also denied any medical problems or medication history, except for controlled gestational hypertension on the fourth patient. Nonetheless, all other caesarean sections on the remaining patients were elective. Table 1 presents a full description of the patients.

Table 1. Patients' surgical and demographic characteristics

Characteristic	Case 1	Case 2	Case 3	Case 4
Age (years)	28	31	34	23
Gestational Age (weeks)	40	37	37	39
Pregnancy Status	G2P1	G2P1	G3P2	G1P0
Diagnosis	- Singleton pregnancy - Prolonged labour - History of IUFD	- Singleton pregnancy - Placenta previa	- Singleton pregnancy	- Singleton pregnancy - Gestational hypertension
Caesarean Section	Emergency	Elective	Elective	Elective
Additional Procedure	None	None	Bilateral Salphingo-oophorectomy	None
SAB Fentanyl Hyperbaric bupivacaine hydrochloride 0.5%	 20 mcg 12 mg	 20 mcg 12 mg	 20 mcg 14 mg	 20 mcg 12 mg
Comorbidity	None	None	None	Gestational hypertension

Abbreviation: SAB: subarachnoid block, IUFD: intra-uterine foetal demise.

All patients received equal standard care according to the routine hospital protocols: (1) six hours of fasting before surgery for elective patients, (2) spinal anaesthesia was performed at the L3-4 or L4-5 level and (3) patients signed the informed consent for anaesthesia, surgery, postoperative QL block procedure and publications.

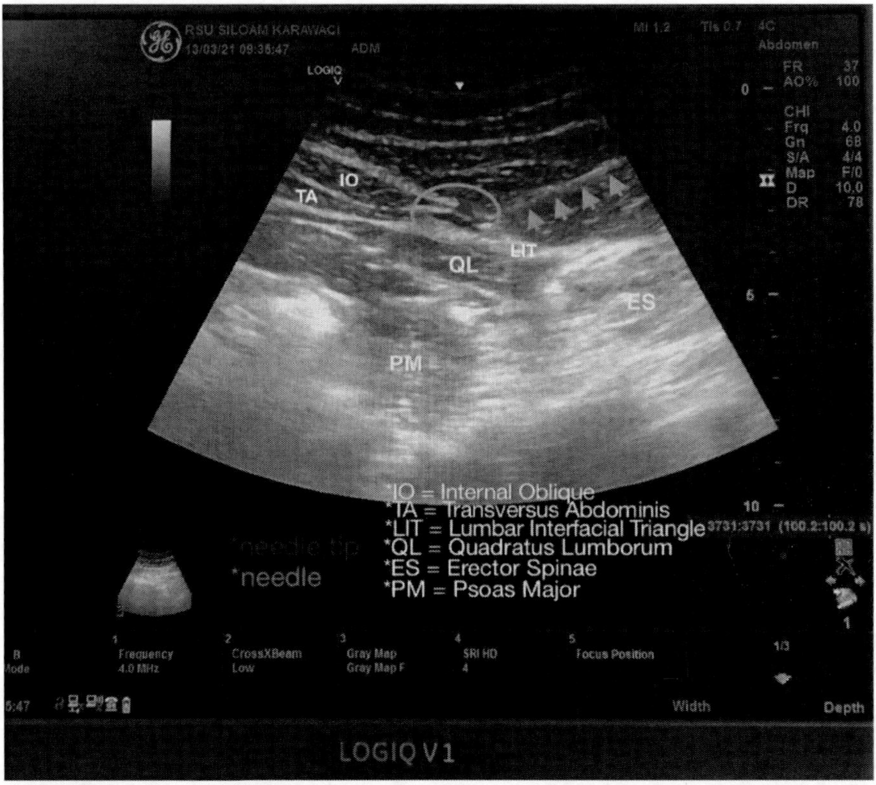

Figure 1. Ultrasound-guided QL block.

After the surgery, the patients were placed in the lateral decubitus position for further skin sterilisation and the ultrasonography-guided QL block. The skin of the posterior flank region was sterilised with a combination of isopropyl alcohol and iodinated povidone. Then, an ultrasound probe was placed at the posterior waist between the costal margin and the iliac crest within the posterior axillary line while simultaneously identifying the external oblique muscle, internal oblique muscle, transversus abdominis muscles, the

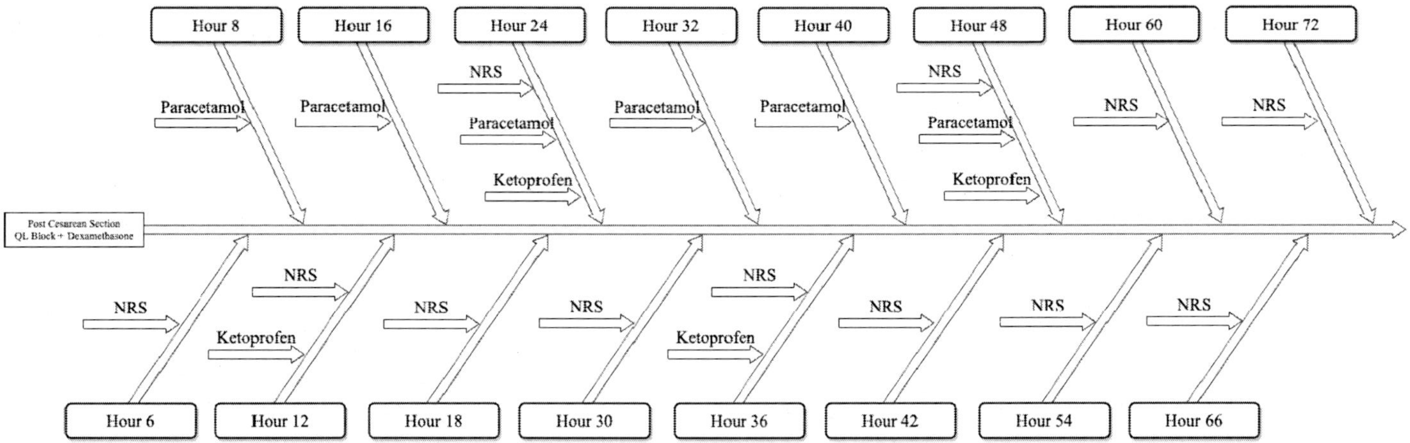

Figure 2. Observation and treatment timeline.

QL muscle, erector spinae muscle, psoas major muscle (shamrock sign) and the aponeurosis of the lumbar interfacial triangle (LIT). After that, the needle was inserted from the posterior with an in-plane approach. The needle tip was positioned until it reached the aponeurosis in the LIT lateral to the QL muscle (QLB2) (Figure 1). Normal saline of three to five millilitres was injected to confirm the position of the needle tip. Isobaric bupivacaine 0.25% 20 ml, lidocaine 2% 5 ml, epinephrine 1:200,000 and dexamethasone 5 mg were injected through a 20 G insulated echogenic needle. A similar procedure was repeated for the contralateral side.

All patients received multimodal analgesia according to a specified timeline (Figure 2). Paracetamol 1,000 mg IV every 8 h and ketoprofen 100 mg Suppository every 12 h were given for the first 48 h postoperatively. Tramadol (50 mg IV) was prescribed if the patient complained of pain at rest with a numeric rating scale (NRS) score $\geq$ 4, and pain on movement with a severity NRS $\geq$ 5. Evaluation of pain was recorded every 6 hours for the first 72 hours after surgery via telephone. Opioid consumption during the first 48 hours was obtained from the integrated medical record from the maternity ward.

Table 2. Pain scale across various postoperative timepoints

Time	**Case 1 NRS**		**Case 2 NRS**		**Case 3 NRS**		**Case 4 NRS**	
	Rest	**Active**	**Rest**	**Active**	**Rest**	**Active**	**Rest**	**Active**
6 hours	5	N/A	3	3	1	2	4	4
12 hours	3	3	3	5	N/A	N/A	3	3
18 hours	2	3	3	5	1	2	1	2
24 hours	1	2	2	5	1	1	1	1
30 hours	1	2	2	4	1	1	N/A	N/A
36 hours	1	2	N/A	N/A	1	1	1	1
42 hours	N/A	N/A	1	3	1	1	1	1
48 hours	1	1	2	4	1	1	1	2
54 hours	1	1	2	3	1	1	3	4
60 hours	1	1	1	2	1	1	3	4
66 hours	1	1	1	2	N/A	N/A	2	4
72 hours	1	1	1	2	1	1	2	4

Abbreviation: NRS: numeric rating scale, N/A: not applicable.

In all four cases, we successfully performed the QL block with the posterior approach. The record of pain assessment using the NRS scale every 6 hours demonstrated that all patients received adequate pain relief up to 72 hours (Table 2). There was no additional tramadol consumption during the first 48 hours after the surgery in any of the patients. No adverse effects, such as local anaesthetic systemic toxicity (LAST), allergic reaction to LA, hypotension, bowel or kidney injury, haematoma or lower-extremity muscle weakness, were noted.

Discussion

The NRS is an effective tool to measure pain intensity, which includes 11 items of whole numbers (0-10 integers), with 0 representing 'no pain' and 10 representing 'worst imaginable pain.' The method of evaluation can be obtained verbally and in our case via telephone, which was suitable, especially during this pandemic period [11]. At rest, an NRS score of 1-3 corresponds to mild pain, 4-6 corresponds to moderate pain and 7-10 indicates severe pain. An NRS score ≤ 4 was considered to be the tolerable pain threshold [12]. On movement, NRS of 1-5 corresponds to mild pain, 6-7 corresponds to moderate pain and 8-10 indicates severe pain [13].

In 2017, Borges et al., found that postoperative pain was present in 92.7% of patients from all 1,062 women undergoing caesarean section [14]. Jadon et al., showed that caesarean section patients who received QL block postoperatively had a significantly lower opioid requirement (0 (1-2)) and pain scores (p = < .0001 and .0024, respectively) [15]. We found similar results in our cases. From our observation, the QL block provided adequate pain relief, with most patients only complaining of mild pain (NRS at rest 1-3 and NRS on movement NRS 1-5) for 72 h postoperatively. The posterior QL block has analgesia coverage at level T7-L1, as Ueshima et al., (2017) described [1, 16]. This coverage may explain why the block we performed on our patients could overcome the post-caesarean pain.

However, the first and fourth patients experienced moderate pain (NRS 5 and 4 at rest) at six hours postoperatively, which might be related to an emergency caesarean section, which the first patient experienced. Akkececi et al., found a relation between patients undergoing emergency caesarean section and more severe postoperative pain and increased need for pain relief [17]. Nevertheless, as the fourth patient's NRS score was four, it was described as tolerable, and no tramadol was given.

We used a combination of bupivacaine, lidocaine, epinephrine and dexamethasone in our study. Bupivacaine is an LA agent with a slow onset of action and a duration of action of approximately two to eight hours [10, 18]. To achieve a rapid onset of action, we combined bupivacaine with lidocaine

[10, 19]. Epinephrine 1:200,000, which was added to lower the risk of systemic toxicity, works by reducing the rate of systemic absorption of the LA [10, 20].

Dexamethasone is known to prolong the duration of LA peripheral nerve block [21]. The precise mechanism of action of perineural dexamethasone is still unknown. However, dexamethasone is said to extend the duration and enhance the quality of regional anaesthesia by causing vasoconstriction, thereby reducing the absorption of LA agents [19, 22]. Kopacz et al., suggested that dexamethasone may also enhance the activation of inhibitory potassium channels in nociceptive C nerve fibres (via glucocorticoid receptors), thereby decreasing the activity of these channels [23]. Chen et al., found that the duration of the blockade is mainly associated with the potency of glucocorticoid activity, which appears to be steroid receptor-dependent and locally mediated [9].

We chose dexamethasone for this study because it has the highest potency related to glucocorticoid activity, as supported by Singariya et al., [24, 25]. Although its usage for perineural administration is considered 'off-label' due to the lack of specific clinical trials regarding its adverse neurotoxicity, many studies have reported no significant increase in serious side effects [26-28]. However, concerns should be addressed to diabetic patients since dexamethasone is known to raise blood glucose levels [29].

There are several approaches to performing the QL block. We chose the posterior approach so that the injection is posterior to the QL muscle (QLB2), where the LA spreads to the paravertebral column, resulting in inhibition of sympathetic nerve fibres present in the thoracolumbar fascia [8,16]. Experts propose that this approach is superior to the lateral approach (QLB1) because of the more predictable paravertebral spread, better visceral pain coverage and lower complications [2, 5, 30, 31].

The limitation of this study is the small sample size and descriptive design. Further studies within a large multi-centre randomised controlled trial are needed to confirm our findings.

Conclusion

In summary, the results showed that QL block with the posterior approach was effective as a part of multimodal analgesia for post-caesarean section pain, and the addition of dexamethasone as an adjuvant provided extended pain relief for up to 72 hours postoperatively.

Competing Interests

The authors declare no conflicts of interest.

Acknowledgments

The study was presented at the 6th International Conference and Exhibition on Indonesian Medical Education and Research Institute (6th ICE on IMERI), Faculty of Medicine, Universitas Indonesia. We appreciate the 6th ICE on the IMERI committee, who had supported the peer review and manuscript preparation before submission to the journal.

References

[1] Huffnagle H J, Norris M C, Leighton B L, Arkoosh V A. Ilioinguinal iliohypogastric nerve blocks--before or after cesarean delivery under spinal anesthesia? *Anesth. Analg*. 1996 Jan;82(1):8-12.

[2] Sebbag I, Qasem F, Dhir S. Bloqueio do quadrado lombar guiado por ultrassom para analgesia pós cesariana: série de casos [Ultrasound guided quadratus lumborum block for analgesia after cesarean delivery: case series]. *Rev. Bras. Anestesiol.* 2017 Jul-Aug;67(4):418-21. Portuguese.

[3] Sutton C D, Carvalho B. Optimal pain management after cesarean delivery. *Anesthesiol. Clin.* 2017 Mar;35(1):107-24.

[4] Blanco R. Tap block under ultrasound guidance: the description of a "no pops" technique. *Reg. Anesth. Pain Med.* 2007;32:130.

[5] Elsharkawy H, El-Boghdadly K, Barrington M. Quadratus lumborum block: anatomical concepts, mechanisms, and techniques. *Anesthesiology.* 2019 Feb;130(2):322-35.

[6] Blanco R, Ansari T, Riad W, Shetty N. Quadratus lumborum block versus transversus abdominis plane block for postoperative pain after cesarean delivery: a randomized controlled trial. *Reg. Anesth. Pain Med.* 2016 Nov/Dec;41(6):757-62.

[7] Blanco R, Ansari T, Girgis E. Quadratus lumborum block for postoperative pain after caesarean section: A randomised controlled trial. *Eur. J. Anaesthesiol.* 2015 Nov;32(11):812-8.

[8] Dhanjal S, Tonder S. Quadratus Lumborum Block. 2021 Aug 23. In: *StatPearls [Internet]. Treasure Island (FL)*: StatPearls Publishing; 2021 Jan–.

[9] Chen Q, An R, Zhou J, Yang B. Clinical analgesic efficacy of dexamethasone as a local anesthetic adjuvant for transversus abdominis plane (TAP) block: A meta-analysis. *PLoS One.* 2018 Jun 14;13(6):e0198923.

[10] Barash P G. Clinical anesthesia. 7th ed. Philadelphia: Wolters Kluwer; 2013.

[11] Hawker G A, Mian S, Kendzerska T, French M. Measures of adult pain: Visual Analog Scale for Pain (VAS Pain), Numeric Rating Scale for Pain (NRS Pain), McGill Pain Questionnaire (MPQ), Short-Form McGill Pain Questionnaire (SF-MPQ), Chronic Pain Grade Scale (CPGS), Short Form-36 Bodily Pain Scale (SF-36 BPS), and Measure of Intermittent and Constant Osteoarthritis Pain (ICOAP). *Arthritis Care Res.* (Hoboken). 2011 Nov;63 Suppl 11:S240-52.

[12] Gerbershagen H J, Rothaug J, Kalkman C J, Meissner W. Determination of moderate-to-severe postoperative pain on the numeric rating scale: a cut-off point analysis applying four different methods. *Br. J. Anaesth.* 2011 Oct;107(4):619-26.

[13] Boonstra A M, Stewart R E, Köke A J, Oosterwijk R F, Swaan J L, Schreurs K M, Schiphorst Preuper HR. Cut-off points for mild, moderate, and severe pain on the Numeric Rating Scale for pain in patients with chronic musculoskeletal pain: variability and influence of sex and catastrophizing. *Front Psychol.* 2016 Sep 30;7:1466.

[14] Borges N C, Costa e Silva B, Pedroso C F, Silva T C, Tatagiba BSF, Pereira LV. Dor pós-operatória em mulheres submetidas à cesariana. *Enferm. Glob.* 2017;16.

[15] Jadon A, Amir M, Sinha N, Chakraborty S, Ahmad A, Mukherjee S. Quadratus Ueshima H, Otake H, Lin J A. Ultrasound-guided quadratus lumborum block: an updated review of anatomy and techniques. *Biomed. Res. Int.* 2017;2017:2752876.

[16] lumborum or transversus abdominis plane block for postoperative analgesia after cesarean: a double-blinded randomized trial. *Braz. J. Anesthesiol.* 2021 Jul 8:S0104-0014(21)00263-3.

[17] Seringec Akkececi N, Oksuz G, Urfalioğlu A, Gunesacar R, Bakacak M, Arslan M, Kelleci BM. Preoperative serum leptin level is associated with preoperative pain threshold and postoperative analgesic consumption in patients undergoing cesarean section. *Med. Princ. Pract.* 2019;28(4):333-40.

[18] Stoelting R. *Pharmacology and physiology in anesthetic practice.* 5th ed. Philadelphia: Wolters Kluwer; 2015.

[19] Shishido H, Kikuchi S, Heckman H, Myers R R. Dexamethasone decreases blood flow in normal nerves and dorsal root ganglia. *Spine* (Phila Pa 1976). 2002 Mar 15;27(6):581-6.

[20] El-Boghdadly K, Pawa A, Chin K J. Local anesthetic systemic toxicity: current perspectives. *Local Reg. Anesth.* 2018 Aug 8;11:35-44.

[21] Marhofer P, Hopkins P M. Dexamethasone in regional anaesthesia: travelling up a blind alley? *Anaesthesia*. 2019 Aug;74(8):969-72.

[22] Attardi B, Takimoto K, Gealy R, Severns C, Levitan E S. Glucocorticoid induced up-regulation of a pituitary K+ channel mRNA in vitro and in vivo. *Recept. Channels.* 1993;1(4):287-93.

[23] Kopacz D J, Lacouture P G, Wu D, Nandy P, Swanton R, Landau C. The dose response and effects of dexamethasone on bupivacaine microcapsules for intercostal blockade (T9 to T11) in healthy volunteers. *Anesth. Analg.* 2003 Feb;96(2):576-82.

[24] Liu D, Ahmet A, Ward L, Krishnamoorthy P, Mandelcorn ED, Leigh R, Brown JP, Cohen A, Kim H. A practical guide to the monitoring and management of the complications of systemic corticosteroid therapy. *Allergy Asthma Clin. Immunol.* 2013 Aug 15;9(1):30.

[25] Singariya G, Choudhary S, Kamal M, Seervi S N, Bihani P, Kumar M. Analgesic sparing effect of dexamethasone with levobupivacaine in quadratus lumborum block in patients undergoing unilateral inguinal hernia repair: A prospective randomised controlled trial. *Indian J. Anaesth.* 2020 Aug;64(8):668-74.

[26] Knight J B, Schott N J, Kentor M L, Williams B A. Neurotoxicity of common peripheral nerve block adjuvants. *Curr. Opin. Anaesthesiol.* 2015 Oct;28(5):598-604.

[27] Kirkham K R, Jacot-Guillarmod A, Albrecht E. Optimal Dose of Perineural Dexamethasone to Prolong Analgesia After Brachial Plexus Blockade: A Systematic Review and Meta-analysis. *Anesth. Analg.* 2018 Jan;126(1):270-9.

[28] Brusich K T. Corticosteroids as adjuvants for peripheral nerve blocks: a mini review. *Int. J. Anaesth. Res.* 2018;1(1)14-7.

[29] Bailard N S, Ortiz J, Flores R A. Additives to local anesthetics for peripheral nerve blocks: Evidence, limitations, and recommendations. *Am. J. Health Syst. Pharm.* 2014 Mar 1;71(5):373-85.

[30] Børglum J, Jensen K, Christensen A F, Hoegberg L C, Johansen S S, Lönnqvist P A, Jansen T. Distribution patterns, dermatomal anesthesia, and ropivacaine serum concentrations after bilateral dual transversus abdominis plane block. *Reg. Anesth. Pain Med.* 2012 May-Jun;37(3):294-301.

[31] Suri A, Sindwani G, Sahu S, Sureka S. Quadratus lumborum block failure: "A must know complication". *Indian J. Anaesth.* 2017 Dec;61(12):1016-8.

Chapter 19

Medical Nutrition Therapy in Clinical Improvement in Tuberculosis and Nasopharyngeal Carcinoma Patients with Refeeding Syndrome: A Case Series

Yohannessa Wulandari*, Novita Salim and Diyah Eka Andayani

Department of Nutrition, Faculty of Medicine, Universitas Indonesia,
Dr. Cipto Mangunkusumo National Hospital, Jakarta, Indonesia

Abstract

Background: Patients with cancer or infectious diseases are vulnerable to malnutrition. Severe malnutrition is a risk factor for refeeding syndrome, a profound shift of fluid and electrolytes that develops from refeeding and causes metabolic disturbances. Low intracellular minerals (hypomagnesemia, hypophosphatemia, hypokalemia), body water imbalance (refeeding oedema), thiamine deficiency, arrhythmia, congestive heart failure and respiratory failure are the signs and symptoms of refeeding syndrome, which can increase morbidity and mortality. *Methods:* We reported four severe malnutrition patients with pulmonary tuberculosis (TB) and nasopharyngeal carcinoma (NPC) who developed refeeding syndrome while being treated for their underlying illness in hospital. Medical nutrition therapy started with energy less than 20 kcal/kgBW/day and increased slowly; low blood electrolytes levels were supplemented with oral or intravenous electrolytes. Patients were

* Corresponding Author's Email: ynessawulandari@gmail.com.

In: The 6th Annual International Conference …
Editors: M. Maidarti, H. Winarto, C. O. M. Jasirwan et al.
ISBN: 978-1-68507-925-3

also given thiamine and another micronutrient supplementation. Patients were monitored closely for clinical conditions, vital signs, water balances and blood electrolyte levels at minimum every 24 hours. *Results:* Before discharge, improvement was seen in clinical signs of refeeding syndrome and blood electrolyte levels. Hospital length of stay was 11 to 27 days. *Conclusion:* Optimal medical nutrition therapy reduces refeeding syndrome severity and improves clinical and blood electrolyte levels.

Keywords: refeeding syndrome, hypophosphatemia, hypomagnesemia, hypokalemia, medical nutrition therapy

Case Series

Introduction

An infectious disease that is often found with malnutrition is tuberculosis (TB). The prevalence in Indonesia shows that 66% of patients with active TB have a body mass index (BMI) below 18.5 kg/m^2 [1]. Another disease that often causes malnutrition is cancer. The prevalence of malnutrition in cancer patients ranges from 20-70% [2]. Nasopharyngeal carcinoma (NPC) is one of the cancers that often causes malnutrition, with a significant decrease in body weight of more than 10% in one month [3].

The goals of medical nutrition therapy in malnourished patients include preventing malnutrition from getting worse and maintaining the nutritional status of the patient. Medical nutrition therapy in malnourished patients begins with screening and determining the degree of malnutrition, as well as screening for the risk of refeeding syndrome, which is often forgotten and undiagnosed. Severe fluid and electrolyte shifts due to refeeding can cause metabolic disorders. Intracellular mineral depletion (hypophosphatemia, hypomagnesemia, hypokalemia), impaired body water ('refeeding oedema'), vitamin B1 (thiamine) deficiency, cardiac arrhythmias, respiratory failure and congestive heart failure are signs and symptoms of refeeding syndrome. Many physiological changes occur during refeeding that can increase patient morbidity and mortality [4].

Information regarding the role of nutritional management on clinical conditions in severely malnourished patients with refeeding syndrome is still very limited and controversial. In this writing, we provide four TB and NPC patients who experienced refeeding syndrome while being treated in hospital. We aim to elevate the consciousness of this syndrome, provide suggestions for preventing refeeding syndrome and outline medical nutrition therapy for clinical improvement, according to the evidence in the literature.

Case 1

A 37-year-old man with pulmonary TB on therapy, community acquired pneumonia (CAP), refeeding syndrome, anemia of chronic disease and prerenal azotemia was admitted because of hypovolemic shock. He had lost 46% of his weight in the last three months, and his BMI was 12.1 kg/m2. On examination, severe deprivation of muscle mass and subcutaneous fat was apparent. On hospital day 2, he was given 44 kcal/kgBW/day of enteral and parenteral nutrition after one month of defeasible food intake. By the next day, potassium plummeted to 2.5 mEq/L. The patient experienced weakness, tachycardia and oedema. Laboratory results showed hyponatremia, hypokalemia, hypophosphatemia, and hypomagnesemia (Table 1). Because of fluid retention and electrolyte imbalances, he was diagnosed with refeeding syndrome. Nutrition therapy started at 19 kcal/kgBW/day and increased 5-10 kcal/kgBW every two days. Oral and intravenous electrolyte supplementation was prescribed. Thiamine 100 mg/day was given. By hospital day 11, signs, symptoms, electrolytes, and other laboratory results had recovered, and the patient was discharged.

Table 1. Electrolyte findings of Case 1

Electrolytes	**Admission**	**Refeeding syndrome (Day 3)**	**Phosphate nadir (Day 5)**	**Before discharge**
Sodium (mEq/L)	127	131	134	138
Potassium (mEq/L)	4	2.5	3	3.9
Chloride (mEq/L)	97	100	105.8	110.7
Phosphate (mg/dL)	0.9	2.6	1.8	2.2
Magnesium (mg/dL)	2.45	1.66	1.57	1.86
Calcium (mg/dL)	7.2	6.5	7.2	7.1

Case 2

A 55-year-old woman with pulmonary TB on therapy, CAP, refeeding syndrome, anemia of chronic disease, drug-induced liver injury and prerenal azotemia was admitted because of severe antituberculosis drug-induced liver injury. She had lost 15% of her weight in the last six months. On admission, severe hyponatremia was corrected intravenously. Her BMI was 15.6 kg/m^2. On examination, there were severe deprivation of muscle mass and subcutaneous fat, and oedema. Nutrition was initiated at 19 kcal/kgBW/day on hospital day 2 after one month of defeasible food intake. On day 4, she was given 28 kcal/kgBW/day. Within the next two days, potassium dropped to 3.3 mEq/L and phosphate to 2.1 mg/dL. She experienced weakness, dyspnea and tachycardia. Laboratory results showed hyponatremia, hypokalemia, hypophosphatemia and hypomagnesemia (Table 2). Nutrition therapy started at 19 kcal/kgBW/day and increased 5-10 kcal/kgBW every two days. She was treated with thiamine 100 mg/day, oral and parenteral electrolyte supplementation. By day 11, signs, symptoms, electrolytes and other laboratory results had recovered, and she was discharged.

Table 2. Electrolyte findings of Case 2

	Admission	**Refeeding syndrome (Day 6)**	**Phosphate nadir (Day 8)**	**Before discharge**
Sodium (mEq/L)	115	133	134	139
Potassium (mEq/L)	5.1	3.3	2.9	3.7
Chloride (mEq/L)	88	101.9	102.7	104.6
Phosphate (mg/dL)	4.5	2.1	1.9	2.1
Magnesium (mg/dL)	1.99	1.87	1.63	1.69
Calcium (mg/dL)	6.7	6.6	6.3	6.3

Case 3

A 52-year-old man with NPC T4N2M0, tracheostomy, cancer pain, CAP, anemia and refeeding syndrome was admitted because of severe pneumonia. He had diminished 29% of body weight in the last six months, and his BMI was 17.3 kg/m2. On examination, the patient had moderate deprivation of muscle mass and subcutaneous fat. On admission, he had mild hyponatremia and hypocalcemia (Table 3). Enteral nutrition began at a level of 12 kcal/kgBW/day after one month of defeasible food intake. Energy intake was increased gradually to 32 kcal/kgBW/day. Within 13 days of admission, he had tachycardia and loss of consciousness. Electrolytes worsened concurrently, hyponatremia, hypokalemia, hypophosphatemia, hypomagnesemia and hypocalcaemia (Table 3). Nutrition therapy started at 15 kcal/kgBW/day and increased 3 kcal/kgBW every two days. After electrolyte correction, he had adequate contact. Thiamine 200 mg/day was given. By hospital day 27, he was discharged with improved clinical conditions.

Table 3. Electrolyte findings of Case 3

Electrolytes	Admission	Refeeding syndrome (Day 13)	Phosphate nadir (Day 14)	Before discharge
Sodium (mEq/L)	129	111	110	132
Potassium (mEq/L)	4.5	3.4	3.3	4.6
Chloride (mEq/L)	103	85	86.9	103
Phosphate (mg/dL)	2.9	1.5	1.4	2.5
Magnesium (mg/dL)	1.79	1.53	1.57	2.23
Calcium ion (mmol/L)	1.05	0.89	0.92	1.08

Case 4

A 63-year-old woman was diagnosed with NPC T3N2M0 on chemoradiation, pulmonary and intracranial metastases, global aphasia, right central seventh nerve paresis, right hemiplegia, CAP, hypertension and refeeding syndrome. Seven days after her first cycle of chemotherapy (5-fluorouracil/cisplatin) and two days after her seventh cycle of radiation, she was admitted to hospital because of loss of consciousness. She had 29% weight loss in the last six months, and her BMI was 16.4 kg/m2. She had had negligible food intake for two weeks. On examination, she had inadequate contact, severe deprivation of

Table 4. Electrolyte findings of Case 4

Electrolytes	Admission	Refeeding syndrome (Day 7)	Phosphate nadir (Day 11)	Before discharge
Sodium (mEq/L)	136	149	138	137
Potassium (mEq/L)	3.2	3.2	2.8	3.3
Chloride (mEq/L)	96.4	110.9	99.8	100
Phosphate (mg/dL)	n/a	3.2	3.1	4.5
Magnesium (mg/dL)	n/a	1.44	1.06	1.39
Calcium ion (mmol/L)	n/a	1.19	n/a	1.13
Calcium (mg/dL)	n/a	9.1	7.6	8.8

muscle mass and subcutaneous fat. Enteral nutrition was initiated on hospital day 3, at a rate of 16 kcal/kgBW/day. On day 6, she was given 43 kcal/kgBW/day. Within the next day, the patient vomited and had dyspnea, tachycardia and congestive heart failure. Laboratory results showed hypokalemia, hypomagnesemia and hypernatremia (Table 4). Nutrition therapy started at 16 kcal/kgBW/day and increased 5-10 kcal/kgBW every two days. Electrolytes were substituted orally and intravenously. Thiamine 100 mg/day was given. By day 25, the patient was discharged with clinical condition improvement.

Discussion

Recognizing patients at refeeding syndrome risk promptly is vital before starting nutritional support. Based on the American Society for Parenteral and Enteral Nutrition (ASPEN) consensus criteria, all patients were at significant risk of refeeding syndrome (Table 5).

Table 5. Risk of Refeeding Syndrome Based on the ASPEN Consensus Criteria

Criteria	**Case 1**	**Case 2**	**Case 3**	**Case 4**
Moderate risk: 2 risk from				
BMI 16–18,5 kg/m^2	-	-	+	+
Weight loss 5% in 1 month	-	-	-	-
None or negligible caloric intake for 5–6 days or <75% of estimated energy requirement for >7 days during acute illness or <75% of estimated energy requirement for >1 month	+	+	+	+
Minimally low prefeeding potassium, phosphate or magnesium levels	-	-	-	+
Evidence of moderate loss of subcutaneous fat	-	-	+	-
Evidence of mild or moderate loss of muscle mass	-	-	+	-
Moderate comorbidities	-	-	-	-
Significant risk: 1 risk from				
BMI <16 kg/m^2	+	+	-	-

Criteria	Case 1	Case 2	Case 3	Case 4
Weight loss 7,5% in 3 months or >10% in 6 months	+	+	+	+
None or negligible caloric intake for > 7 days or < 50% of estimated energy requirement for > 5 days during acute illness or < 50% of estimated energy requirement for > 1 month	+	+	+	+
Moderately/significantly low prefeeding potassium, phosphate or magnesium levels	+	-	-	-
Evidence of severe loss of subcutaneous fat	+	+	-	+
Evidence of severe loss of muscle mass	+	+	-	+
Severe comorbidities	+	+	+	+

ASPEN, American Society for Parenteral and Enteral Nutrition; BMI, body mass index. +/- denotes presence/absence of a risk factor.

All patients had tachycardia and no arrhythmias. In the fourth case, there was vomiting, shortness of breath and heart failure. The first case had refeeding syndrome after one day of energy administration of 44 kcal/kgBW/day. The second case experienced refeeding syndrome after four days of initial energy administration of 19 kcal/kgBW/day and two days after energy was increased to 28 kcal/kgBW/day, which suggests that administering a higher amount of energy causes a more rapid refeeding syndrome. The first case was also at very high risk for refeeding syndrome due to a BMI less than 14 kg/m^2 and severe hypophosphatemia prior to nutrition. As TB patients with severe malnutrition were found to have a higher mortality rate, it is recommended to provide high-calorie nutritional supplementation. However, the initiation of nutrition in severely malnourished patients carries a risk of triggering the refeeding syndrome. Until now, epidemiological data related to refeeding syndrome in TB are still very limited. A study in Chhattisgarh, India by Chebrolu et al., [5] investigated the risk of refeeding syndrome in severely malnourished TB patients. On energy intake, it was found that 37% of patients experienced refeeding syndrome, especially hypophosphatemia. However, the sample of this study is relatively small, so epidemiological data regarding TB patients with refeeding syndrome in larger studies and other areas are still needed.

The third case had a decrease in consciousness and electrolyte levels when energy 32 kcal/kgBW/day was given. The fourth case experienced refeeding syndrome after four days of initial energy administration of 16 kcal/kgBW/day and one day after energy was increased to 43 kcal/kgBW/day. Information about refeeding syndrome in NPC patients is still limited. In a study by Gonzales et al., [6] in Mexico, the incidence of refeeding syndrome in cancer patients receiving enteral or parenteral nutrition was reported to be 24.5%. Head and neck cancer patients are susceptible to this syndrome. A report from Denmark showed a 20% incidence of refeeding syndrome in head and neck cancer patients (n = 54) [7]. Similarly, from a cohort study in the Netherlands, patients with sepsis and malignancy (n = 178) were at higher risk of developing refeeding syndrome. Malnutrition due to disease is reported in around half of oncology patients and is related to poor outcomes. Previous electrolyte abnormalities are also frequently found in head and neck cancer patients. These are paraneoplastic and are usually related to regimens or other ingredients in chemotherapy. Hypophosphatemia is common in sepsis patients, mostly because of gram-negative bacteria, and its severity relates to disease severity. Hypokalemia can also occur because of antibiotic therapy. In addition, antibiotics containing sodium can cause fluid retention. Consequently, it is also difficult or maybe impossible to attribute absolute clinical and biochemical complications to one or more causative variables. These abnormalities often happen together and reinforce each other rather than as a single cause of refeeding syndrome [8].

The main treatment for patients who have experienced refeeding syndrome is electrolyte correction followed by nutrition with the principle of lowering energy or increasing energy slowly [9]. Medical nutrition therapy for all cases started with energy 19, 19, 12 and 16 kcal/kgBW/day, respectively. The energy given to the first, second and fourth cases was increased gradually by 5-10 kcal/kgBW every two days. In the third case, energy was increased more slowly by 3 kcal/kg every two days. Initiation of energy administration in all patients was in accordance with the ASPEN 2020 recommendation for patients at significant risk of refeeding syndrome, which was 10-20 kcal/kgBW/day, then gradually increased by 33% every 1-2 days. Patients at risk for refeeding syndrome should include close electrolyte monitoring and electrolyte correction as appropriate before initial feeding. Patients with low electrolyte levels prior to nutrition should be given aggressive supplementation [9].

Several factors must be taken into consideration when starting and increasing energy intake, including physiological responses (e.g., cardiac rhythm and changes in serum electrolytes) and initial feeding tolerance. Numerous of the accessible suggestions are common and unclear, giving recommendations such as increasing at a slow pace, [10] gradually progressing [11] or providing a fair increase in calorie [12] and achieving target requirement within 3-7 days [13]. In a review article, McCray et al., [14] recommended early feeding of 200-300 calories every 3-4 days. However, these recommendations are based solely on clinical events. Others suggest supplementing electrolytes and expanding energy by adding 10-15 mmol of phosphate for every 1,000 calories provided [12].

O'Connor et al., [15] systematically checked accessible research and determined that malnutrition was a more vital marker while recognizing risky patients than the first total calories given. Nonetheless, concurring to the available writing, nutrition ought to be started at 50% of the estimated basal energy expenditure. It is generally suggested that energy needs start at 10 kcal/kgBW/day [16]. A more conservative method of feeding ought to be considered to determine whether the patient is critically ill and suffering from malnutrition. Energy should be initiated to at least 5 kcal/kgBW/day [16, 17]. This should be increased slowly over the next seven days to reach a total requirement of 25-35 kcal/kg/day [18].

Boateng et al., [16] suggested a gradual energy increase from day 4-10 to achieve a total calorie intake of 15-20 kcal/kgBW/day. The choice to extend or diminish energy supply ought to be based on symptoms and biochemical observation [16]. McClave et al., [19] recommended feeding starting at 10 kcal/kgBW/day and increasing at a slow pace. The goal is to achieve 20 kcal/kgBW/day in the first 10 days then to target 25-35 kcal/kgBW/day, according to recommendations for head and neck cancer patients [19].

Research by Vignaud et al., [20] revealed that severely malnourished patients who were given higher energy (23.2 ± 5 kcal/kgBW/day) on the first day had refeeding syndrome and all died from complications of multiorgan failure or acute respiratory distress syndrome (ARDS) with fluid and electrolyte imbalances [20]. Doig et al., [21] in their randomized trial pointed out that refeeding syndrome patients who were given low energy (maximum 20 kcal/kgBW/day) in the first two days showed clinical improvement, higher survival rates, and lower days of treatment and mortality than in patients given standard energy. In all cases, the refeeding syndrome was managed with an initial energy of less than 20 kcal/kgBW/day that was gradually increased, a correction of low electrolytes and thiamine supplementation. All patients showed improvement in symptoms and signs of refeeding syndrome, length of stay for 11 days, 11 days, 27 days and 25 days. They were discharged with improvement in laboratory results and blood electrolyte levels.

Thiamine supplementation was given to all patients. In patients with refeeding syndrome, the National Institute for Health and Care Excellence (NICE) recommends giving thiamine 200-300 mg/day for 10 days [22]. Friedli et al., [23] recommended administering thiamine at 200-300 mg/day for 1-5 days. ASPEN recommends thiamine supplementation at 100 mg/day for 5-7 days [9]. The first and second cases received thiamine 100 mg/day for six days. The third case was given thiamine 200 mg/day for 21 days. The fourth case received thiamine 100 mg/day for 10 days. The daily thiamine requirement according to the recommended dietary allowance (RDA) is 1.1 mg for adult men, 1.2 mg for adult women and 1.4 mg for pregnant and lactating women [24]. The WHO recommends giving thiamine for mild deficiency of 10 mg/day orally for one week, followed by oral thiamine 3-5 mg/day for a minimum six weeks. For severe thiamine deficiency, intravenous thiamine 50-100 mg then 10 mg/day intramuscularly for one week, followed by oral thiamine 3-5 mg/day for at least six weeks [25]. In the four case series patients, no side effects occurred during thiamine supplementation.

Conclusion

Refeeding syndrome is difficult to diagnose (underdiagnosed), causing avoidable morbidity in at-risk patient groups. Initiation of energy administration in all patients was decreased at the time of refeeding syndrome and then increased slowly. All low blood electrolyte levels were corrected enterally and intravenously. Thiamine supplementation was given to all patients. Initial assessment with malnutrition risk screening, including refeeding syndrome risk screening, is vital. Before providing nutrition to at-risk patients, electrolytes must be examined. Thiamine is given at the beginning of treatment. Giving calories slowly, especially in the first week, becomes important until the patient is metabolically stable ('start low go slow'). Special attention was given to laboratory tests, and electrolyte level examinations should be performed daily. Once the refeeding syndrome has occurred, we should reduce the energy intake, aggressively correct the electrolyte abnormalities and give vitamin B supplementation. Routine blood phosphate and magnesium levels examination in at-risk patients. Phosphates are often excluded from chemical panel tests unless specifically requested so that phosphates are often referred to as 'forgotten electrolytes.' Better multidisciplinary cooperation is needed in dealing with severely malnourished patients admitted to hospital. Patients who are severely malnourished or at risk of malnutrition and refeeding syndrome should be treated by a nutritional therapy team.

Competing Interests

None declared.

Acknowledgments

The authors wish to thank Dr Sri Sukmaniah, MSc, SpGK(K), Dr Ida Gunawan, MS, SpGK(K) and Dr Diana Sunardi, M. Gizi, SpGK (Department of Nutrition, Universitas Indonesia) for all inputs, comments, sharing and support. The authors obtained no specific grant from any funding agency in the public, commercial or not-for-profit sectors.

This article was presented at the 6th International Conference and Exhibition on Indonesian Medical Education and Research Institute (6th ICE on IMERI), Faculty of Medicine, Universitas Indonesia. We thank the 6th ICE on the IMERI committee, who had supported the peer-review and manuscript preparation before submitting it to the journal.

References

[1] Amin Z, Bahar A. Tuberkulosis paru. In: Sudoyo W A, Alwi I, Simadibrata M, Setiati S, eds. Buku ajar ilmu penyakit dalam, 6th ed. Jakarta: Pusat Penerbitan Departemen Ilmu Penyakit Dalam Fakultas Kedokteran Universitas Indonesia; p. 863–82.

[2] Arends J, Baracos V, Bertz H, Bozzetti F, Calder P C, Deutz NEP, et al. ESPEN expert group recommendations for action against cancer-related malnutrition. *Clin. Nutr.* 2017; 36(5):1187–96.

[3] Irungu C W, Oburra H O, Ochola B. Prevalence and predictors of malnutrition in nasopharyngeal carcinoma. *Clin. Med. Insights Ear Nose Throat.* 2015;8:19–22.

[4] Menteri Kesehatan Republik Indonesia. Keputusan Menteri Kesehatan Republik Indonesia Nomor Hk.01.07/Menkes/393/2019 tentang pedoman nasional pelayanan kedokteran tata laksana malnutrisi pada dewasa. Kementerian Kesehatan RI; 2019.

Accessed 2021 Jun 10. Available on: https://galihendradita.files.wordpress.com/2021/06/2019-pnpk-malnutrisi.pdf.

[5] Chebrolu P, Laux T, Chowdhury S, Seth B, Ranade P, Goswami J, et al. The risk of refeeding syndrome among severely malnourished tuberculosis patients in Chhattisgarh, India. *Indian J. Tuberc.* 2020;67(2):152–8.

[6] González Avila G, Fajardo Rodríguez A, González Figueroa E. The incidence of the refeeding syndrome in cancer patients who receive artificial nutritional treatment. *Nutr. Hosp.* 1996;11(2):98–101.

[7] Rasmussen S O, Kristensen M B, Wessel I, Andersen J R. Incidence and risk factors of refeeding syndrome in head and neck cancer patients-an observational study. *Nutr. Cancer.* 2016;68(8):1320–9.

[8] Windpessl M, Mayrbaeurl B, Baldinger C, Tiefenthaller G, Prischl FC, Wallner M, et al. Refeeding syndrome in oncology: report of four cases. *World J. Oncol.* 2017;8(1):25–9.

[9] da Silva J S V, Seres D S, Sabino K, Adams S C, Berdahl G J, Citty S W, et al. ASPEN consensus recommendations for refeeding syndrome. *Nutr. Clin. Pract.* 2020;35(2):178–95.

[10] Kiraly L N, McClave S A, Neel D, Evans D C, Martindale RG, Hurt RT. Physician nutrition education. *Nutr. Clin. Pract.* 2014;29(3):332–7.

[11] Friedli N, Stanga Z, Sobotka L, Culkin A, Kondrup J, Laviano A, et al. Revisiting the refeeding syndrome: results of a systematic review. *Nutrition.* 2017;35:151–60.

[12] Solomon S M, Kirby D F. The refeeding syndrome: a review. *J. Parenter. Enter Nutr.* 1990;14(1):90–7.

[13] Kraft M D, Btaiche I F, Sacks G S. Review of the refeeding syndrome. *Nutr. Clin. Pract*. 2005;20(6):625–33.

[14] McCray S, Parrish C R. Refeeding the malnourished patient: lessons learned. *Pract. Gastroenterol.* 2016;155:56–66.

[15] O'Connor G, Nicholls D. Refeeding hypophosphatemia in adolescents with anorexia nervosa: a systematic review. *Nutr. Clin. Pract.* 2013;28(3):358–64.

[16] Boateng A A, Sriram K, Meguid M M, Crook M. Refeeding syndrome: treatment considerations based on collective analysis of literature case reports. *Nutrition.* 2010;26(2):156–67.

[17] Viana Lde A, Burgos MG, Silva Rde A. Refeeding syndrome: clinical and nutritional relevance. *Arq. Bras. Cir. Dig.* 2012;25(1):56–9.

[18] Centers for Disease Control and Prevention. Lactic acidosis traced to thiamine deficiency related to nationwide shortage of multivitamins for total parenteral nutrition -- United States, 1997. *MMWR Morb. Mortal. Wkly Rep.* 1997 Jun 13;46(23):523–8.

[19] McClave S A, Taylor B E, Martindale R G, Warren M M, Johnson D R, Braunschweig C, et al. Guidelines for the provision and assessment of nutrition support therapy in the adult critically ill patient: Society of Critical Care Medicine (SCCM) and American Society for Parenteral and Enteral Nutrition (A.S.P.E.N.). *J. Parenter. Enteral Nutr.* 2016;40(2):159–211.

[20] Vignaud M, Constantin J M, Ruivard M, Villemeyre-Plane M, Futier E, Bazin J E, et al. Refeeding syndrome influences outcome of anorexia nervosa patients in intensive care unit: an observational study. *Crit. Care.* 2010;14(5):R172.

[21] Doig G S, Simpson F, Heighes P T, Bellomo R, Chesher D, Caterson I D, et al. Restricted versus continued standard caloric intake during the management of refeeding syndrome in critically ill adults: a randomised, parallel-group, multicentre, single-blind controlled trial. *Lancet Respir Med.* 2015;3(12):943–52.

[22] National Collaborating Centre for Acute Care (UK). Nutrition support for adults: oral nutrition support, enteral tube feeding and parenteral nutrition. *London: National Collaborating Centre for Acute Care (UK);* 2006. Accessed 2020 Jun 12. Available on: www.rcseng.ac.uk.

[23] Friedli N, Stanga Z, Culkin A, Crook M, Laviano A, Sobotka L, et al. Management and prevention of refeeding syndrome in medical inpatients: an evidence-based and consensus-supported algorithm. *Nutrition.* 2018;20(47):13–20.

[24] Frank L L. Thiamin in Clinical Practice. *JPEN J Parenter. Enteral. Nutr.* 2015 Jul;39(5):503-20.

[25] World Health Organization. Thiamine deficiency and its prevention and control in major emergencies. Geneva: *World Health Organization;* 1999. Accessed 2020 Jun 19. Available on: https://apps.who.int/iris/handle/10665/66139.

Chapter 20

Use of Non-Steroidal Anti-Inflammatory Drugs (NSAIDS) to Decrease Inflammation in Mild-to-Moderate COVID-19 Patients

Ronald Winardi Kartika[1,*], Marcel Tendean[1], Bernard[2], Katarina[2] and Em Yunir[3]

[1]Faculty of Medicine, Krida Wacana Christian University, Jakarta, Indonesia
[2]Ukrida Hospital, Jakarta, Indonesia
[3]Faculty of Medicine Universitas Indonesia,
Cipto Mangunkusumo Hospital, Jakarta, Indonesia

Abstract

Background: Non-steroidal anti-inflammatory drugs (NSAIDs) are one of the most used drugs and have a wide range of uses. Previous research has debated the use of NSAIDs against the increased risk of side effects when used in patients with acute respiratory infections, including COVID-19. Several studies have used corticosteroids as anti-inflammatory agents for COVID-19. Corticosteroids have the potential to treat COVID-19, but their administration is controversial due to limited clinical evidence. Recommendations from the World Health Organization (WHO) suggest avoiding the use of corticosteroids in COVID-19 patients with comorbid autoimmune disease. This review assesses the effect of NSAID and/or corticosteroid use in mild-to-moderate COVID-19 patients. *Research Methods:* Retrospective analysis of medical records. The inclusion criteria of patients were mild-to-moderate COVID-19 symptoms who received NSAID or steroid therapy.

---

* Corresponding Author's Email: ronald.kartika@ukrida.ac.id.

In: The 6th Annual International Conference …
Editors: M. Maidarti, H. Winarto, C. O. M. Jasirwan et al.
ISBN: 978-1-68507-925-3

As an indicator of the usefulness of anti-inflammatory therapy (antipyretics are clinical and laboratory inflammation such as leukocytes, neutrophil/monocyte ratio, erythrocyte sedimentation rate (ESR) and C-reactive protein (CRP). This study was conducted at UKRIDA Hospital from January to June 2021 and has passed the ethical review from FKIK UKRIDA with submission No.: 1052/SLKE-IM/UKKW/FKIK/KE/II/ 2021 *Results:* There were 246 mild-to-moderate cases of COVID-19 with more male research subjects than women (62.6%: 37.4%). The use of NSAIDs, steroids and combinations of NSAIDs + steroids is almost equal (35.4%: 30.1%: 34.5%). The most common NSAIDs used were colchicine (16.3%), paracetamol (12.2%), ibuprofen (9.3%), cox-3 (8.7%) and metamizole (3.5%). In the steroid group, most used methylprednisolone (54.1%) compared to dexamethasone (45.9%). Results from the Kruskal–Wallis statistical test showed that the combination of NSAIDs and corticosteroids compared to individual NSAID and corticosteroid use can reduce inflammation markers Leucocytes, p = .035; N/L ratio, p = .049; ESR, p = .046; and CRP, p = .028. *Conclusion:* The use of a combination of NSAIDs and steroids in COVID-19 patients can significantly reduce inflammatory markers compared to NSAIDs or corticosteroids alone. The use of NSAIDs in COVID-19 patients is safe and does not prolong hospitalization.

Keywords: non-steroid anti-inflammatory drugs, steroid, COVID-19

Case Series

Coronavirus infection (COVID-19) is a cause of morbidity and mortality worldwide, including in Indonesia. Many trials are underway, but little is currently known about a therapy that can cure the COVID-19 infection. Non-steroidal anti-inflammatory drugs (NSAIDs) are inexpensive and widely available with anti-inflammatory properties that are useful as adjunctive therapy to increase the cure rate for COVID-19 patients. The therapeutic use of NSAIDs in treating COVID-19 of various levels (mild, moderate and severe) has been widely used, but further research and clinical trials are needed to ensure safety and efficacy [1].

NSAIDs are a group of drugs used to reduce inflammation, thereby relieving pain and reducing fever. In dealing with pain, NSAIDs work by inhibiting inflammation-triggering hormones, namely prostaglandins. With reduced inflammation, pain and fever will also decrease [2].

In response to the many questions to the European Medicine Agency (EMA) regarding the issue of NSAIDs, especially ibuprofen, which can worsen the coronavirus disease. There is currently no scientific evidence establishing a link between ibuprofen and worsening of COVID-19 complications. The EMA is monitoring the situation closely and will review any new information that becomes available on this issue in the context of the pandemic. It is still debated the use of NSAIDs in the treatment of COVID-19 [3].

The EMA recommends that when starting the treatment of fever or pain in COVID-19 patients, patients and healthcare professionals should consider all available treatment options, including paracetamol and NSAIDs. Most ibuprofen-containing medicines are authorised at national level, as a painkiller and in some countries also as an antipyretic (fever medicine). Each drug has its own benefits and risks, which can be seen in each product information and follow the European National Medicine Guidelines, which mostly recommend paracetamol as first-line treatment for fever and pain. Other NSAIDs (such as ibuprofen, colchicine, COX2 inhibitor) might be used as an anti-inflammatory therapy in respiratory infection [4].

Further to the review conducted by the EMA Safety Committee on the safety of ibuprofen and ketoprofen, the EMA emphasised the need for timely epidemiological studies to provide adequate evidence of the effect of NSAIDs on COVID-19 prognosis [5].

Anti-pain therapy usually involves giving NSAIDs (such as aspirin, ibuprofen and meloxicam), paracetamol, opioid drugs (methadone, morphine or codeine) or adjunctive drugs to help relieve pain while COVID-19 patients are being treated. During the pandemic, anti-inflammatory drugs were also used in the treatment of COVID-19. A study between 17 January and 10 August 2020 in Scotland, Wales and England with 78,674 cases stated that 4,211 patients used systemic NSAIDs prior to hospital admission [6].

NSAIDs are among the most commonly used drugs and have a wide range of uses. NSAIDs include nonselective cyclooxygenase (COX) inhibitor (such as ibuprofen, aspirin (acetylsalicylate), diclofenac and naproxen), as well as selective COX2 inhibitor (such as celecoxib, rofecoxib, etoricoxib, etoricoxib, lumoracoxib and valecox) [7].

Concerns have been raised that NSAIDs may increase the risk of side effects when used in patients with acute respiratory infections, including COVID-19. Several studies have used corticosteroids as anti-inflammatory agents in COVID-19. Steroids have the potential to treat COVID-19, but their administration is still controversial due to limited clinical evidence. The WHO recommends avoiding the use of corticosteroids for COVID-19, but the Surviving Sepsis Campaign recommends their use in COVID-19 patients with acute respiratory distress syndrome (ARDS). Another study by Granei, in 2021, reported that low-dose prednisolone was superior to other regimens in shortening the length of hospital stay in patients with moderate to severe COVID-19 [8].

This review assesses the effects of NSAIDs and steroids in mild to moderate COVID-19 patients, including those with ARDS.

Hypothesis: NSAID antipyretics are safe and effective as mild-to-moderate COVID-19 anti-inflammatory drugs.

Research Benefits: Contribution to medical care about safe and effective anti-inflammatory treatment for the COVID-19 virus infection.

Research novelty: The standard of anti-inflammatory therapy as an antipyretic in COVID-19 patients is still needed for evidence-based medicine to be reported in Scopus accredited journals.

General Purpose

1. To determine the anti-inflammatory effects of NSAIDs (paracetamol or ibuprofen, colchicine or metamizole or COX-2 inhibitor) and steroids (Methyl Prednisolone or Dexamethasone).
2. To see the safety of NSAID drugs as a complementary therapy to standard COVID-19 therapy according to the Ministry of Health.
3. To see the anti-inflammatory effect of NSAIDs compared to steroids in COVID-19 therapy.

Specific Purpose

1. To see changes in leukocytes as an anti-inflammatory effect of NSAIDs in COVID-19 therapy.
2. To see changes in the N/L Ratio as an anti-inflammatory effect of NSAIDs in COVID-19 therapy.

Research Methods

This cohort study used consecutive sampling from the medical records of COVID-19 patients treated at UKRIDA Hospital from January to June 2021. The methods are retrospective data based on clinical findings.

The population of this study was COVID-19 patients treated at UKRIDA Hospital during a certain period with criteria inclusion of mild-to-moderate COVID-19, and sampling was carried out at least two times, once when in the ER and once when leaving the hospital. Exclusion criteria were patients with incomplete medical record data.

Results

Table 1 shows the distribution of COVID-19 patients in terms of severity of illness.

Table 1. COVID-19 patients in UKRIDA Hospital in January-June 2021 based on classification

COVID-19 Criteria	**N**	**Percentage (%)**
Mild	116	47.2
Moderate	130	52.8
Total	246	100

Table 2. Criteria of mild-moderate COVID-19 patients in UKRIDA Hospital January-June 2021

Mild-Moderate COVID-19	**n**	**Percentage (%)**
Age		
≤ 30	51	20.7
31-40	47	19.1
41-50	42	17.0
51-60	57	23.2
61-70	31	12.6
71-80	18	7.3
Gender		
Male	154	62.6
Female	92	37.4
Therapy		
NSAID (paracetamol, ibuprofen, colchicine, Metamizole, COX2 inhibitor)	87	35.4
Steroid (methylprednisolone, dexamethasone)	74	30.1
Combination (NSAID + steroid)	85	34.5
Total	246	100

Table 2 shows that almost all adult patients have the same risk of getting COVID-19, but that patents aged 51-60 years are more likely to be hospitalised at UKRIDA hospital. Males have a higher risk compared to females (62.4%: 37.4%). The percentage of COVID-19 patients who were treated with NSAIDs or steroids or a combination of NSAIDs + steroids was almost the same (35.4%: 30.1%: 34.5%).

Table 3 shows the kind of NSAIDs used in mild-to-moderate COVID-19 patients in UKRIDA Hospital. Paracetamol is the most frequently used NSAID as anti-inflammation therapy in COVID-19 patient who has fever and pain.

Table 3. The use of NSAIDs in mild-to-moderate COVID-19 patients in UKRIDA Hospital

NSAID	N	Percentage (%)
Paracetamol (single)	82	33.3
Ibuprofen (single)	19	7.7
Colchicine (single)	33	13.4
COX2 inhibitor (single)	26	10.7
Metamizole (single)	6	2.4
Combination of 2 NSAIDs	49	19.9
Combination of > 2 NSAIDs	31	12.6
Total	246	100

Table 4 shows the kind of steroids used to treat mild-to-moderate COVID-19 patients at UKRIDA Hospital. Both methylprednisolone and dexamethasone are steroids used for anti-inflammation therapy.

Table 4. The use of steroids in mild-to-moderate COVID-19 patients in UKRIDA Hospital

NSAID	N	Percentage (%)
Methylprednisolone	40	54.1
Dexamethasone	34	45.9
Total	74	100

Table 5 shows that a combination of NSAIDs + steroid decreased the markers of inflammation significantly compared with just NSAIDs or steroids.

Table 5. Comparison of NSAIDs, steroids, and combination of NSAID + steroid with Delta Leucocyte in mild-to-moderate COVID-19 patients

Inflammation Marker	**NSAID n = 87**	**Steroid n = 74**	**NSAID+Steroid n = 85**	***P***
Δ Leucocyte	-450.0 (-8900.0–7440.0)	1325.0 (-8100.0–6520.0)	-1100 (-9950–5980)	.035
Δ Ratio N/L	-1.08 (-7.28–41.10)	-0.39 (-7.44–7.02)	-0.61 (-6.00–4.66)	.049
Δ ESR	-5.74 (-100.0–46.4)	-3.9 (-99.3–60.9)	-14.0 (-56.4–22.6)	.046
Δ CRP	-14.2 (-152.9–84.31)	-9.8 (-136.0–21.6)	-19.0 (-73.1–4.2)	.028

[*] Median (min-max), Mann-Whitney test.

Discussion

This study used several NSAIDs in addition to steroid therapy as anti-inflammatory treatment, which became standard in the treatment of COVID-19 at UKRIDA Hospital. This study used colchicine, paracetamol, ibuprofen, COX2 inhibitor and metamizole as NSAIDs. Colchicine is considered suitable for COVID-19 because it is well known for its immunomodulatory properties in severe auto-inflammatory diseases; it is very effective in the treatment of gout because of its strong anti-inflammatory effect [9, 10].

One of the early symptoms of COVID-19 is fever due to the increased inflammation process. This fever can be accompanied by more dominant respiratory symptoms such as shortness of breath, cough and difficulty swallowing, and anosmia (a condition when a person cannot smell odours). In this case, all drugs approved for this indication can be used, although paracetamol is often used as an NSAID that functions as an antipyretic and anti-inflammatory. We also used metamizole as an antipyretic and anti-inflammatory agent in mild-to-moderate COVID-19 patients. Metamizole is often used as adjunctive therapy for COVID-19 patients as an analgesic and antipyretic to treat the most common symptoms of COVID-19, which are fever and diffuse pain. However, the use of metamizole is banned in some countries because of the rare side effects that include neutropenia and agranulocytosis. So far, there have been no safety reports of metamizole in COVID-19 patients. For short-term hospital use, metamizole appears to be a safe choice when compared to other widely used analgesics. However, a mid- and long-term safety assessment of metamizole is still needed [11].

This study also used ibuprofen as an NSAID. Several previous studies have reported that taking ibuprofen as an anti-inflammatory did not worsen the infection with the coronavirus that causes COVID-19 [12, 13]. Other studies have mentioned the dangers of giving ibuprofen to SARS-CoV2 infection at the start of the pandemic because ibuprofen can worsen the condition of COVID-19 patients. A recent study by Wong found that ibuprofen did not increase the severity of the disease. This article provides clear evidence that NSAIDs are safe to use in COVID-19 patients [5, 14].

Information relating the use of NSAIDs, such as ibuprofen, with the occurrence of COVID-19 severity is still uncertain with clinical data in humans and is being discussed by other state authorities, such as the EMA, US FDA and WHO [14, 15].

In this COVID-19 therapeutic study, patients who received colchicine had lower levels of inflammatory markers such as D-dimer and serum levels of C-reactive protein (CRP) compared to patients who did not receive colchicine. COVID-19 therapy with colchicine provides a potential synergistic effect of the cytokine cascade at various levels. Colchicine inhibits the inflammatory pathway by inhibiting the inflammasome NLRP3, microtubule-based inflammatory cell chemotaxis, leukotriene and cytokine production, and phagocytosis. An accumulation of colchicine in white blood cells will reduce motility, loosen adhesion and chemotaxis, and inhibit superoxide anion formation and mast cell degranulation [15].

This study found a decrease in inflammation with a decrease in leukocytes, N/L ratio, ESR and serum C-reactive protein (CRP). There was a significant decrease of all these markers in the NSAID + steroid combination group compared to the separate NSAID or steroid groups ($p = .035$, $p = .049$, $p = .046$, $p = .028$).

For years, intensivists have searched for easily quantifiable and readily available parameters that might reflect the intensity of systemic stress and/or inflammation in critically ill patients following shock, multiple trauma, major surgery or sepsis. The ratio of neutrophil count to lymphocyte count is a quick and simple parameter of systemic inflammation and stress in critically ill [17].

Other laboratory tests that are most commonly used to assess inflammation are the erythrocyte sedimentation rate (ESR) and serum C-reactive protein (CRP). Research in the field of rheumatology shows a positive correlation and moderate relationship between CRP and ESR in the flare phase of rheumatoid arthritis or in acute inflammation [18, 19].

COVID-19 patients with mild-to-moderate criteria who received NSAID + steroid combination therapy had a shorter length of stay than those who received NSAID or steroids alone. This article also finds that the use of combination NSAIDs and Corticosteroids in COVID-19 therapy is safe and does not aggravate COVID-19 symptoms.

Conclusion

The use of NSAIDs in combination with steroids used as anti-inflammatory agents in COVID-19 can reduce inflammatory markers.

C-reactive protein is a significant marker of inflammation that has a correlation with the cure rate of COVID-19 patients with mild-to-moderate symptoms.

Competing Interests

There is no conflict of interest in this study.

Acknowledgments

The study was funded by Universitas Indonesia. This article was presented in the 6th International Conference and Exhibition on Indonesian Medical Education and Research Institute (6th ICE on IMERI), Faculty of Medicine, Universitas Indonesia. We thank the 6th ICE on IMERI committee, who had supported the peer-review and manuscript preparation for publication to Nova Science Publishers, Inc.

References

[1] Arshad Ali S, Baloch M, Ahmed N, Arshad Ali A, Iqbal A. The outbreak of Coronavirus Disease 2019 (COVID-19)-An emerging global health threat. *J. Infect. Public Health.* 2020 Apr;13(4):644-6.

[2] Mehta P, McAuley D F, Brown M, Sanchez E, Tattersall R S, Manson J J; HLH Across Speciality Collaboration, UK. COVID-19: consider cytokine storm syndromes and immunosuppression. *Lancet*. 2020 Mar 28;395(10229):1033-4.

[3] Qin C, Zhou L, Hu Z, Zhang S, Yang S, Tao Y, Xie C, Ma K, Shang K, Wang W, Tian D S. Dysregulation of immune response in patients with Coronavirus 2019 (COVID-19) in Wuhan, China. *Clin. Infect. Dis.* 2020 Jul 28;71(15):762-8.

[4] Nieto-Torres J L, Verdiá-Báguena C, Jimenez-Guardeño J M, Regla-Nava J A, Castaño-Rodriguez C, Fernandez-Delgado R, Torres J, Aguilella V M, Enjuanes L. Severe acute respiratory syndrome coronavirus E protein transports calcium ions and activates the NLRP3 inflammasome. *Virology*. 2015 Nov;485:330-9.

[5] Wong A Y, MacKenna B, Morton C E, Schultze A, Walker A J, Bhaskaran K, et al.; OpenSAFELY Collaborative. Use of non-steroidal anti-inflammatory drugs and risk of death from COVID-19: an OpenSAFELY cohort analysis based on two cohorts. *Ann. Rheum. Dis*. 2021 Jul;80(7):943-51.

[6] Castaño-Rodriguez C, Honrubia J M, Gutiérrez-Álvarez J, DeDiego M L, Nieto-Torres J L, Jimenez-Guardeño J M, Regla-Nava J A, Fernandez-Delgado R, Verdia-Báguena C, Queralt-Martín M, Kochan G, Perlman S, Aguilella V M, Sola I, Enjuanes L. Role of Severe Acute Respiratory Syndrome Coronavirus Viroporins E, 3a, and 8a in replication and pathogenesis. *mBio*. 2018 May 22;9(3):e02325-17.

[7] Little P. Non-steroidal anti-inflammatory drugs and COVID-19. *BMJ*. 2020 Mar 27;368.

[8] Karamanou M, Tsoucalas G, Pantos K, Androutsos G. Isolating colchicine in 19th century: an old drug revisited. *Curr. Pharm. Des*. 2018;24(6):654-8.

[9] Imazio M, Brucato A, Adler Y. A randomized trial of colchicine for acute pericarditis. *N. Engl. J. Med*. 2014 Feb 20;370(8):781.

[10] Nidorf S M, Thompson P L. Why colchicine should be considered for secondary prevention of atherosclerosis: an overview. *Clin. Ther*. 2019 Jan;41(1):41-8.

[11] Martínez G J, Robertson S, Barraclough J, Xia Q, Mallat Z, Bursill C, Celermajer D S, Patel S. Colchicine acutely suppresses local cardiac production of inflammatory cytokines in patients with an acute coronary syndrome. *J. Am. Heart Assoc*. 2015 Aug 24;4(8):e002128.

[12] Cocchi E, Chiale F, Gianoglio B, Deorsola L, Pace Napoleone C, Fagioli F, Peruzzi L. Colchicine: an impressive effect on posttransplant capillary leak syndrome and renal failure. *Pediatrics*. 2019 May;143(5):e20182820.

[13] Cao B, Wang Y, Wen D, Liu W, Wang J, Fan G, et al. A Trial of Lopinavir-Ritonavir in Adults Hospitalized with Severe COVID-19. *N. Engl. J. Med*. 2020 May 7;382(19):1787-99.

[14] Deftereos S G, Giannopoulos G, Vrachatis D A, Siasos G D, Giotaki S G, Gargalianos P, et al. Effect of colchicine vs standard care on cardiac and inflammatory biomarkers and clinical outcomes in patients hospitalized with Coronavirus Disease 2019: The GRECCO-19 Randomized Clinical Trial. *JAMA Netw. Open*. 2020 Jun 1;3(6):e2013136.

[15] Dupuis J, Sirois M G, Rhéaume E, Nguyen Q T, Clavet-Lanthier M É, Brand G, Mihalache-Avram T, Théberge-Julien G, Charpentier D, Rhainds D, Neagoe P E, Tardif J C. Colchicine reduces lung injury in experimental acute respiratory distress syndrome. *PLoS One*. 2020 Dec 2;15(12):e0242318.

[16] Nonaka D, Takase H, Machii M, Ohno K. Colchicine therapy for deep vein thrombosis in a patient with vascular-type Behçet disease: A case report. *Medicine* (Baltimore). 2020 Apr;99(16):e19814.

[17] Scarsi M, Piantoni S, Colombo E, Airó P, Richini D, Miclini M, et al. Association between treatment with colchicine and improved survival in a single-centre cohort

of adult hospitalised patients with COVID-19 pneumonia and acute respiratory distress syndrome. *Ann. Rheum. Dis*. 2020 Oct;79(10):1286-9.

[18] Montealegre-Gómez G, Garavito E, Gómez-López A, Rojas-Villarraga A, Parra-Medina R. Colchicine: A potential therapeutic tool against COVID-19. Experience of 5 patients. *Reumatol. Clin*. (Engl Ed). 2021 Aug-Sep;17(7):371-5.

[19] Montealegre-Gómez G, Garavito E, Gómez-López A, Rojas-Villarraga A, Parra-Medina R. Colchicine: A potential therapeutic tool against COVID-19. Experience of 5 patients. *Reumatol. Clin*. (Engl Ed). 2021 Aug-Sep;17(7):371-5.

[20] Merad M, Martin J C. Pathological inflammation in patients with COVID-19: a key role for monocytes and macrophages. *Nat. Rev. Immunol*. 2020 Jun;20(6):355-62.

[21] Banu N, Panikar S S, Leal L R, Leal A R. Protective role of ACE2 and its downregulation in SARS-CoV-2 infection leading to Macrophage Activation Syndrome: Therapeutic implications. *Life Sci*. 2020 Sep 1;256:117905.

Organizing Committee

Advisory Board	Ari Fahrial Syam Badriul Hegar
Steering Committee	Dwiana Ocviyanti Anis Karuniawati Rahyussalim Budi Wiweko Diantha Soemantri Trinovita Andraini
General Chair	Mila Maidarti
Vice Chair	Isabella Kurnia Liem
Scientific Editorial Boards	Hariyono Winarto Chyntia Olivia Maurine Jasirwan Eka Dian Safitri Virna Dwi Oktariana
Editorial Asistants	Fiona Esmeralda Nur Eulis Pujiastuti Nahdiyat Aly Lamuri Daniel Martin Simadibrata Naivedh Bhat
Academic Writer	Karomah Widianingsih
Administrator	Indina Tarziah

Editor Contact Information

Dr. Mila Maidarti, SpOG K-FER, PhD
Chairperson
The 6th ICE on IMERI
Faculty of Medicine, Universitas Indonesia
Jalan Salemba Raya No. 6, Central Jakarta, Indonesia
Email: Imeri-ic@ui.ac.id

Dr. Hariyono Winarto, SpOG (K)
Gynecologist, Oncologist
Faculty of Medicine Universitas Indonesia,
Dr. Ciptomangunkusumo Hospital, Jakarta, Indonesia
Email: hariyono.winarto@ui.ac.id

Dr. Chyntia Olivia Maurine Jasirwan, PhD, SpPD, KGEH, FINASIM
Faculty, Consultant
Gastroenterology and Hepatology
The Department of Internal Medicine, Medicine Universitas Indonesia,
Jakarta, Indonesia
Email: chynmadu@gmail.com

Dr. Eka Dian Safitri, Sp.THT-KL
The Center of Clinical Epidemiology and Evidence-Based Medicine FMUI
Dr. Cipto Mangunkusumo General Hospital
Salemba, Jakarta, Indonesia
Email: ed_safitri@yahoo.com

Dr. Virna Dwi Oktariana S.PM (K)
Head of Glaucoma Division
The Department of Ophthalmology, Faculty of Medicine
Universitas Indonesia, Jakarta, Indonesia
Email: virnadwi_dr@yahoo.com

Index

E

F

G

H

I

K

L

M

N

O

P

Q

R

S

T

U

V

W